Cracking The Dementia Code

Cracking The Dementia Code

Creative solutions
to cope with changed behaviours

Karen Tyrell, CDP, CPCA

First Published in Canada 2013 by Influence Publishing

© Copyright Karen Tyrell, CDP, CPCA
All rights reserved. No part of this publication may be reproduced, stored in or introduced into a retrieval system, or transmitted, in any form, or by any means (electronic, mechanical, photocopying, recording or otherwise) without the prior written permission of the publisher. This book is sold subject to the condition that it shall not, by way of trade or otherwise, be lent, resold, hired out, or otherwise circulated without the publishers prior consent in any form of binding or cover other than that in which it is published and without a similar condition including this condition being imposed on the subsequent purchaser.

Book Cover Design: Adam Mountstevens
Typesetting: Greg Salisbury
Author Photographer: Judith Laurel

DISCLAIMER: This book has been created to inform individuals with an interest in Dementia & Alzheimer's disease. It is not intended in any way to replace other professional health care or mental health advice, but to support it. Readers of this publication agree that neither Karen Tyrell nor her publisher will be held responsible or liable for damages that may be alleged or resulting, directly, or indirectly, from their use of this publication. All external links are provided as a resource only and are not guaranteed to remain active for any length of time. Neither the publisher nor the author can be held accountable for the information provided by, or actions resulting from accessing these resources.

Story of the Cover Photo

It is almost impossible to find the right words to express my gratitude to Dawn Thomas and her family for providing the perfect photo for the front cover of my first published book. No Hallmark card could ever adequately express my appreciation for their assistance. When attempting to choose from a variety of stock photo actors to place on the front cover of this book, I just could not seem to find anything that adequately illustrated my deep message and vision. Then, miraculously, an answer evolved just as naturally as other solutions relevant to the book-writing process have done. Fate has had everything to do with it. Along came my friend Dawn with a special family photo.

Dawn was my first Recreation Manager in a long-term care home in Ontario, when I was just starting out in the dementia care field. We have remained friends even though our journeys have taken us to opposite ends of Canada. Dawn has been caring for her mother with Alzheimer's disease for almost two years. She recently wrote about her caregiving experiences in The Digby County Courier, her local newspaper. To help you to understand her situation, here is a copy of her article in that paper:

"My mother spent many winter days in a cold rink. We would be on the road for skating lessons long before and after the school bell rang. My brother's hockey meant she would travel and spend weekends in other area rinks. It didn't stop there. Like most mothers, she was busy with our piano lessons, homework, high school struggles and three pets at any given time.

My mother taught Sunday school, sang in the choir, baked homemade bread and cared for the largest strawberry patch in all of Bear River. She also made many of our clothes. She sewed costumes, curtains, quilts and stuffed toys.

As I go through similar motions with my own daughter, without nearly as much enthusiasm and even less patience, I realize the dedication she had and sacrifices she made as a mother. She told me that would happen.

I recently popped by my mother's sewing room to cut the fabric for my window valances. She let me pick the material from her neatly folded collection. We were surrounded by family photos, baskets of thread and trays of drying lavender.

She decided to make us some tea. I heard a crash and a swear word. When I got to the kitchen, I saw a look of exasperation. "What did I come in here for?" she asked. Alzheimer's disease takes simple memories and skills away from my mother. There are a lot of complicated steps to making tea now. Operating a kettle and stove top has become a risk to her safety.

As we made the tea together, I spotted her pills on the table, hidden in the flower prints of the placemat. I poured her some water and handed her the small pile of pills. "I need something to eat with them," she says. One hour and forty distractions later, we sat down to tea. My valances would wait.

My role as a daughter keeps changing. Our lives are coming full circle. We stay afloat while we constantly juggle this reversal, still trying to preserve the uniqueness that makes her a mother and me a daughter."

I thank Dawn and her mother Geraldine Morine for allowing me to share their mother/daughter photo with the readers of this book. In addition, I would like to include a special mention and thank you to Dawn's close friend and Digby County Courier reporter, Jonathan Riley, for using his talents to create such a fantastic photo! It is heart-warming and pleasurable to know that a special and fun day for all of you produced such a great keepsake. I am wholeheartedly grateful. My sincerest thanks!

This book is dedicated to all those who have been and will be affected by dementia—particularly the caregivers.

Testimonials

"Karen's passion and dedication towards helping those affected by dementia is remarkable. Her practical tips and methods will certainly benefit all caregivers who read it."
Dr. Justin Davis, Scientific Director, nognz brain fitness

"A simple, but thorough, guide to understanding Dementia and Alzheimer's disease and how to manage behaviours with dignity and grace."
Wendy Scott, RN, Owner of Nurse Next Door, Burnaby/New Westminster/Tri-Cities

"Karen is a very knowledgeable trainer and resource person. She is a talented, highly skilled professional who goes the extra mile. The training session I attended was excellent, well paced, and very practical. She continues to offer support and advice. Thank you, Karen for all your assistance."
Valerie Ostara, Clinical Hypnotherapist

"Karen Tyrell above all is a compassionate and dedicated healthcare specialist. Working with Alzheimer patients and their families is her calling. She is an effective communicator, sharing her skills through the Certified Dementia Practitioner training program and her "Cracking the Dementia Code" presentations. Karen continually displays a rare combination of integrity and professionalism while maintaining a great sense of humour. I fully support her and am pleased to offer my endorsement."
Mike Oakley, Owner of Home James Services for Seniors

"Karen's simple, caring and calming approach to dementia care is an inspiration to all those caring for individuals with dementia. She is passionate about sharing her knowledge and helping others to make this often difficult journey as positive as it can be."
Julie Bernard, BTR, Recreation Therapist, West Vancouver Adult Day Centre

"Karen demonstrates keen insight and experience into behaviours relative to dementia. Her course content and teaching on this topic are sound and instructional—Karen makes learning fun and engaging. Karen is truly passionate about her work with families and people with dementia."
Cheryl Guenther, CDP, General Manager, The Royale-Pacifica Resort Retirement Residence/Leisureworld Seniors Care Corporation

"Karen Tyrell's "Cracking the Dementia Code" provides clear, easy-to-understand information about dementia. Using situations gleaned from the experiences of the participants, Karen demonstrates how to deal with difficult behaviour brought on by dementia. "Cracking the Dementia Code" is beneficial for anyone living or working with people with dementia. Family members and professionals can learn new techniques to improve their skills and the lives of those living with dementia."
Margaret Hansen, Coordinator of Volunteers, New Vista Care Centre

Acknowledgements

First and foremost, I want to acknowledge a wonderful selfless man named Douglas Tyrell, my father, who loved his children so much that his devotion instilled in me the desire to constantly make him proud during and after his life on earth.

I am very grateful for my family. I would like to thank my mothers Lorraine and Irma, and my siblings Kelly, Chris, and Angela (and their families) for providing continual love and support even as the physical distance between us grew. I love you all dearly!

Several amazing close friends have entered my life at different stages and have been by my side for many years. I know that we will continue to share many great memories as we carry on along our paths. For this, I feel blessed.

It would not be possible to be where I am today if not for Barrie Fraser, my devoted life partner. Not only has he been accepting and supportive of my dreams, goals, and work commitments, but he continually encourages me to delve into the realm of curiosity and self-improvement. Over the years he has cultivated in me a higher level of thinking in a way I never knew existed by opening my eyes to a bigger picture of life.

I must acknowledge my amazing friend Bonnie Wannamaker for all her assistance in helping me create my company in order for me to continue to keep my passion as my profession. She coached me even though we were no longer in the same province and taught me about the world of business and assisted me with the essentials. I will always be grateful for her eternally optimistic confidence in me and in my abilities. Without this encouragement from her and her guru entrepreneurial partner Terry Telford, I would not have gathered the courage to take the initial leap on my journey as a Dementia Consultant and Educator.

I would like to give a big "thank you" to all the amazing nurses, care aids, and managers I've worked with in long-term care homes over the years. I extend special mention to Dawn Thomas, Lisa Herjavec, and June Giles who are magnificent teachers and continue to be incredible supporters. With tongue in cheek, I thank those who I perceived, at times, to be looking at me as if I needed my head examined! Each of you sparked the fire by motivating me to stand firm and believe in my inner convictions while I continued my attempts to manage dementia related behaviours with alternative approaches. Thank you for the magnificent motivation!

I strongly believe that my passion would not exist today if not for witnessing the challenges resulting from inadequate approaches and methods for managing dementia related behaviours in long-term care homes. In my opinion, many of these occasions were related to the lack of dementia training provided, practiced, and promoted.

For all the incredible family members I have met and assisted on my journey thus far, I am pleased to have known you. Your overwhelming appreciation has given me the desire and hunger to keep going. In particular, I want to thank Mr. Elliott Parker for allowing me to be at his side during and after his caregiving journey. He has taught me so much about the inner world of being a family caregiver.

I would like to express my gratitude for all the wonderful people I have met in my life over the years. Each individual has impacted my achievements and contributed towards my accomplishments. One connection has led me to another, and another, and so forth. For example, Mike Oakley of Home James Service for Seniors Inc. introduced me to Sonya Eskoy from Virtual Ink Writing and Editing Services who motivated and supported me to initiate this book. I will always be thankful to them both! More recently, while assisting me with marketing questions, it was Christine Till, The Marketing Mentress, who led me to her publisher, Julie Salisbury and Influence Publishing.

I truly believe the connections I have made over the years have led me to this pinnacle moment in my life. I know that Julie and her team from Influence Publishing have come together to assist me in sharing my dementia knowledge with families and caregivers all over the world. Warmest thanks to all!

Author Prologue

Alzheimer's disease and other types of dementias are harsh realities that exist in our world today. Writing from experience, I believe it is time for major changes to take place in the medical care and management of those afflicted with dementia. A paradigm shift needs to take place that focuses on non-pharmacological interventions as a first line of defence for dealing with the challenging behaviours that often accompany dementia related disease. This book is written to contribute to the needed change.

Concurrently, the information in this book should not be treated as medical advice. While the ideas expressed are designed as a resource for all interested persons and to help alleviate stress for caregivers, results cannot be guaranteed, including improvement of the loved one's symptoms. The ideas in this book are an approach to treatment, and are not to be considered a treatment alternative for dementia. It remains important to obtain appropriate medical advice and to ask questions and communicate openly with medical care providers.

The Cracking the Dementia Code™ workshop has provided the basic material to write this book (also called Cracking the Dementia Code). The book is intended to extend the content of the workshop to a wider audience as well as to be used as a reference for workshop participants. It is meant to assist both family caregivers and professional caregivers (those who work in long-term care, retirement homes, day programs, home care, and other services). The book provides an easy-to-follow understanding of the core concepts of creative non-drug approaches and therapies that have been used by many others and myself for many years.

This book is structured to allow readers to gradually develop a new mindset by opening their potential towards new and creative understandings by reducing the need for pharmaceutical treatments for as long as possible in order to manage behaviours associated with dementia. This exciting journey accelerates in chapter four.

Chapter one sets the stage for caregivers and opens the mind to the range of possible expectations a caregiver may encounter. It also offers practical ways to address common caregiving challenges.

Chapter two concentrates on positive proactive outlooks with helpful suggestions on ways to maintain a healthy brain.

Chapter three is full of resources about dementia both reversible and non-reversible. It also has lots of details about Alzheimer's disease, the most common cause of dementia.

The exciting journey of understanding and addressing dementia related behaviours in your caregiving role begins in chapter four. It is with hope that the concepts shared in this book will provide the reader with either a light bulb moment, or a boost to move to a different level of thinking. Perhaps readers will be reassured that what you thought was the right approach is the right approach. Or, perhaps readers may feel more appreciated for the wonderful work they have been doing.

To demonstrate a selection of the creative concepts present in this book; chapter eleven 'Meaning Behind the Behaviour—Putting It Into Practice' includes true stories mainly from long-term care settings that may provide readers with insight into the practical use of creative solutions to manage behaviours of others in later stages of dementia.

Chapter thirteen focuses on hopes for the future including a call for Canada to join other countries with a National Alzheimer Strategy.

Throughout the book you will find boxes of **Helpful Hints** to highlight important information. In addition, you will find periodic reminders of the importance to take deep breaths.

If you are a family or professional caregiver pressed for time, know that you are welcome to navigate to chapter four 'Behaviours and Coping Possibilities' as we fully understand the importance of time and getting right into the "meat and potatoes" of how to address challenging behaviours.

How and why helping those affected by dementia has become a major part of my life...

Since I can remember, I've always been passionate about helping others. My business, Personalized Dementia Solutions, allows me to pursue this passion by offering personalized assistance to those affected by Alzheimer's and other dementia related diseases. Let me take you back to when and why I started my journey, and how I became a Dementia Consultant and Educator.

When I was about ten years old, I saw an elderly woman walking past my house with her hands full of groceries. As I watched her walk to the end of my street, I could see that she was really struggling. I decided to run out and offer her my assistance to get home; she was positively pleased! I will never forget the high I felt that day and it inspired me to start regularly helping others.

Around this time, I can recall my father and I discussing my potential career options. I remember envisioning that I would like to be a nurse. I recall telling him that I wanted to be the kind of nurse that makes people smile. So it was decided—I would become a nurse. When I was in junior high, we were required to dissect things such as large crickets and frogs; let's just say I became a little squeamish. Realizing I did not have the strongest stomach led me to question my plan to become a nurse; however, I still knew I wanted to help others.

Around the end of my high school years, I decided to volunteer at my local hospital to test my future career path. This was before mandatory high school volunteer hours were introduced. The Volunteer Coordinator at the hospital asked me about my skills and interests and recommended the Health Records Department. While I did enjoy the data entry and organizational aspects of the job, there just wasn't enough human interaction for me. I returned to the Volunteer Coordinator, hoping to find a position that suited me better; she suggested the Radiology Department. I absolutely loved it! It was so interesting to work with the imaging computers. I also thoroughly enjoyed meeting new people every day and making them feel comfortable in the waiting areas.

After high school, it was time to reassess what I loved about my role in the Radiology Department. It wasn't so much the X-ray machines that I enjoyed, but rather being there for the people. I liked welcoming them, answering their questions, and providing them guidance and comfort. Surely, I didn't have to be in the Radiology Department to do that! So, I did a little more soul searching and realized that the people I enjoyed working with the most were the elderly patients. The next step was easy; I decided to volunteer at a local long-term care home to determine if this could be my new career path.

On my first day at the nursing home, I was a little nervous. As we were preparing to play a game of sandbags, my supervisor left me alone with about ten of the residents. They were all sitting in a circle looking either bored or curious about me. I felt awkward just standing there. Instead of waiting for my supervisor to return, I began to introduce myself and request names. Thereafter, I decided to make a game of it and started acting silly, pretending it was hard work to remember all of their names. The residents laughed and I felt a strong feeling of belonging and connection. At that moment, in the middle of that circle, I knew this was the career for me.

Since there was no program called "Making Seniors Smile," I did some investigating. A college program available in the mid 1990's, leading to a diploma in Activation Coordinator/Gerontology caught my interest. This two-year program consisted of three days of recreation theory and two days of working with seniors as part of the course placement each week.

As I studied the common conditions that affect the elderly, such as Alzheimer's disease (a progressive brain disease common in people over the age of 65) and other dementia related diseases (these will be discussed in chapter three), I became aware of many discrepancies. I realized that the proper care practices and environments I was learning about in the theory class did not match the reality of what was happening in the long-term care home where my practicum placement was taking place. In my opinion, the conditions were less than ideal.

For example, after providing an afternoon of quality programs in the Alzheimer unit, there were a few residents who did not want me to leave. While attempting to gently leave, I did what I could to promise them that I would return later. Unfortunately, the only way out was through a set of glass doors in the middle or common area of the unit. My heart broke because the affected residents were able to see me walking away and began to pound on the other side of the locked doors, pleading for me to take them with me. I will never forget that day.

Returning to school in the year 2000 to complete another two-year diploma program called Social Service Worker/Gerontology, I chose the local Alzheimer's Society (Leeds-Grenville chapter in Ontario) for my college placement. Once this work placement was complete, I was invited to become a Board Member. Around the same time, I had the good fortune to obtain a full-time job as a Recreation Assistant with a long-term care home. After about two years on the Board, I was nominated for the role as President and held this position for four years. During this time, the Board and staff members of this Alzheimer's Society joined forces to propel our dreams into changes that would help families and individuals in the community cope with the disease.

In 2006, my role with the Alzheimer Society changed as the opportunity to become the Executive Director for the chapter arose. I remained in this role for two and a half years before moving to British Columbia in June 2009.

While in this executive role, a role that I enjoyed greatly, a number of limitations bothered me. For example, our office was only open Monday to Friday from 9:00 am to 5:00 pm. The Alzheimer Society received messages on evenings and weekends from family caregivers requiring support and it bothered me that we couldn't answer in a more timely fashion. We also were not permitted to make home visits. As many caregivers could not leave their loved ones alone at home to come into the office to get the support they so desperately needed, the inability of our staff to make home visits was a real problem. In these cases, conversations over the phone were all we could offer. Further, in some cases, phone calls became an issue as the caregiver had to be careful what to say while their loved one was in the room with them. I found all these limitations frustrating, as did the staff members at the Alzheimer's Society. How could we do more to help? How could I do more to help?

A more recent chapter of my life...

Upon arriving in British Columbia in 2009, the frustrations for myself and others involved in dementia services identified during my time with the Alzheimer's Society (in Ontario) and over 14 years in total of working in various care settings, remained one of my dominant passions as well as my desire to help those affected. This passion would not go away. Shortly after settling in to my new home in BC, I began working once again in a long-term care home as a Recreation Assistant. I soon realized similar discrepancies and limitations in dementia care in BC as had been apparent in Ontario. In addition, I noticed there were really no obvious differences in the overall level of dementia knowledge available to those providing dementia services in the two provinces.

In addition to my work as a Recreation Assistant, I also signed up to be a volunteer Support Group Facilitator to assist caregivers in my community. It soon became evident to me there was a lack of, or shortage of, services and support not only in my community but also in most communities across BC. In this volunteer role, I found that many of the family members I interacted with were not aware of alternative non-drug approaches or unique strategies to manage dementia behaviours. In some ways it makes sense—why would they know all these helpful strategies? In many cases, those I supported were having their first experience with someone afflicted with dementia. There were many times I felt like jumping out of my chair to offer all kinds of helpful suggestions. On the other hand, I knew this type of advocacy was not an expectation appropriate to my volunteer Support Group Facilitator role.

Considering my past experiences working in long-term care homes and frustrations surrounding the limitations experienced at the community level, I decided I needed to take action in my new home province of British Columbia. I made a strong commitment at the end of 2009; I decided it was time to take action by making my passion into my profession to provide assistance to struggling families in a personalized way by starting my own business. I have set up Personalized Dementia Solutions to provide support to families and caregivers that will best suit their schedules. In addition, I have created and designed workshops and other services that allow me to share my cumulative knowledge with my clients about personalized alternative behavioural and non-drug approaches.

My passion for education and helping families…

In the beginning, caring for someone with a progressive dementia, including Alzheimer's disease, may not be difficult. However, as time passes and if the person begins to exhibit odd or strange behaviours this could become frustrating and add to the stress level of the caregiver.

While working in long-term care settings over the years, I had the privilege of coming up with creative ideas to manage many of the common behaviours that arose in the residents with dementia. Every day, I found myself using innovative strategies to ease the fear, concerns, anxiety, and agitation of the residents living at my workplaces. How could I teach others about these creative strategies?

At that time, courses were lacking for front line staff regarding using non-pharmaceutical (or reduced levels of pharmaceuticals) along with behavioural related approaches as a first defence in the treatment of Alzheimer's and other related dementias.

Understanding dementia and how to address the common behaviours is also so important for family caregivers because it can prevent caregiver burnout. "Knowledge is Power," as Sir Frances Bacon (1561 – 1626) once quoted. Therefore, I created a fun interactive workshop called, Cracking the Dementia Code™ to present and teach new angles and creative approaches that may lead to better understandings of the behaviours commonly associated with Alzheimer's disease and related dementias. These creative non-drug approaches are easy to learn and can be used by anyone.

It is important for individuals diagnosed with dementia living in long-term care homes to have their caregivers understand the full range of options at their disposal. Armed with this knowledge, caregivers will have the necessary tools to offer the proper care and approaches that best suit the present stage of their dementia.

Whether you are a family member or a paid caregiver, I hope you realize that you are very important and much needed. I also hope you will find this book helpful as you move forward on your caregiving journey.

Warm regards,
Karen Tyrell, CDP, CPCA
Personalized Dementia Solutions

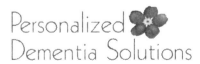

Phone: 778-789-1496
E-mail: info@dementiasolutions.ca
Website: www.DementiaSolutions.ca

Table of Contents

Story of the Cover photo
Dedication
Testimonials
Acknowledgements
Author Prologue
Contents

Chapter 1: Caring for You, the Caregiver 1
    Caregiver Burnout 3
    Asking for Help 5
    Self-Care 9
    Long Distance Caregiving 12
    Changing Relationships 15

Chapter 2: Proactive Ways to Maintain a Healthy Brain 19
    Cognitive Reserve 20
    Exercising the Brain (Neuroplasticity) 21
    Brain Health 22
    Six Key Pillars of a Brain Healthy Lifestyle 23
    Exercise the Whole Brain 26
    Hearing Loss and Brain Health 29

Chapter 3: Understanding Dementia and Alzheimer's 33
    What really is Dementia? 33
    Changes in Terms Used in the Medical World 37
    Symptoms of Dementia 37
    Common Causes of Dementia: Reversible/Treatable 39
    Causes of Dementia: Non-Reversible 44
    What is Alzheimer's Disease? 50
    Signs and Symptoms of Alzheimer's Disease 52
    Stages of Alzheimer's Disease 56
    The "Memory Onion" Analogy 60
    Emotional Memory 61
    More In-Depth Information and Background 62
    Dr. Aloysius "Alois" Alzheimer 62

Types of Alzheimer's Disease 63
Risk Factors for Alzheimer's disease 64
Genetics 65
Current Research 67
Medications 69

Chapter 4: Behaviours and Coping Possibilities 71
What is Behaviour? 72
Possible Behaviours You May Experience 72
Conflict 73
Coping Possibilities 75

Chapter 5: The Dementia Code 85
Manage With Tact, Flattery, and Artifice 86
Why Manage Behaviours? 89
How to Crack the Dementia Code 90
The Power of Asking "Why?" 92

Chapter 6: Gathering the Ph.A.C.T.S.™ 95
Becoming a Detective 95
Enhancing Learning: Case Study 102

Chapter 7: Cracking Down and Getting Creative 105
Creative Non-Drug Therapies 105

Chapter 8: Therapeutic Reasoning™ 117
Keeping the Peace 118
Putting Therapeutic Reasoning™ to Practice 121
Case Study Solutions 125

Chapter 9: Approach, Approach, Approach! 129
Gentle Approaches 129
Person Centred Approach 130
Importance of Knowing the Person You are Caring for 132
Consistent Routines 134

Chapter 10: Importance of Good Communication 135
Non-Verbal Communication 136
Tips for Effective Communication 137
Ways to Address Conflict 139

Chapter 11: Meaning Behind the Behaviour 141

Chapter 12: Being Proactive 159
When is it Time for Professional Support? 159
When a Caregiver Can No Longer Manage the Care 160
Planning Ahead 164

Chapter 13: Hopes for the Future 165
The Future of Dementia Related Care in Canada 166
Future of Dementia Related Care around the World 168

Conclusion 171
Citations 175

Chapter 1

Caring for You, the Caregiver

"When we give cheerfully and accept gratefully, everyone is blessed."
Maya Angelou

Caring for someone with Alzheimer's disease and/or other related dementias (ADRD) is not always easy. The acronym ADRD will be used regularly to refer to Alzheimer's disease and other related dementias throughout the remainder of this book.

As a family member, it may be difficult for you to realize that your role as daughter/son/wife/husband has now changed. Your previous relationship may have suddenly evolved into a role called 'Caregiver.' For many this is not an easy transition. Seeing your loved one change can be heartbreaking.

Caregiving can be very rewarding; it may also be stressful and challenging, regardless of whether you are a family member or a paid caregiver. Many of you already know this. The role may also be unacknowledged by others, including the person you are caring for. Before we go any further, I want to say 'Thank you!' You certainly deserve to hear this. Thank you for all you do; you are truly making a difference.

Being a caregiver (whether or not you have fully accepted your new role as such) will teach you many things about yourself and your capabilities. It can also take a toll on your physical, emotional and mental health.

This stress may take many forms. For instance, you may feel exhausted, frustrated, and angry taking care of someone who regularly exhibits difficult behaviours. As a family caregiver you may also feel guilty because you would like to be able to do more or provide better care, despite all the great things that you already are doing. Perhaps you are starting to feel lonely because all the time you spend caregiving has affected your social life.

I can't stress this enough—it is critical that you make the time to take care of yourself and that you know when to reach out to others for help. This is because I worry about you and your wellbeing including your stress level. Based upon what I have learned about stress over the past few decades, stress can really make us sick.

> **Helpful Hint:** Being a sick caregiver is not good for anyone!

Throughout this book, I want to assist you in getting through the stressful times. To do so, it is best to first understand stress and how it may be controlled. Before we begin, I invite you to take a deep breath.

Stress is a fact of life. It is the way we respond to stress that can have a negative effect on us. According to the Canadian Mental Health Association (CMHA), stress is defined as any change to which we have to adapt. Their website states, "By understanding ourselves and our reactions to stress-provoking situations, we can learn to handle stress more effectively." Many events may trigger a stress response including both positive and negative changes, as well as internal and external stressors that take shape as real or perceived threats. Not all stress is bad. Yet, the effects of chronic stress tend to build up over time.

Ultimately, if you are stressed, your body will respond by altering the secretions of certain hormones and chemicals. Dr. David B. Samadi explains in his article "Surprising Ways Stress Affects Your Whole Body" published by Foxnews.com "Cortisol, the primary stress hormone, inhibits functions that are a detriment to the 'fight-or-flight' response. Specifically, it alters the immune system response and suppresses the digestive tract, reproductive system and growth processes." If your immune system is not working properly then it may not be able to fend off invaders or infections in the body. Physical symptoms that may arise due to stress include migraines, ulcers, muscle tension, fatigue, sleep problems, obesity, memory impairment, worsening of skin problems, irritability, and depression. According to the CMHA, Canadian researchers found that chronic stress more than doubled the risk of heart attacks. Different people may feel stress in different ways. Being a sick caregiver is not good for anyone!

So how can we control our stress? According to the CMHA, the goal of managing stress is to signal the "relaxation response" inside your body. Breathing is one effective way to communicate with your body to inform it that you are relaxed and not feeling stressed. Good breathing habits will improve both your psychological and physical well-being. Exercise is another excellent way to reduce stress and cortisol levels, according to Dr. David B. Samadi. Learning several effective ways that work for you to cope with stress will help to ease your body and your mind. Yet, as a first step, you need to fully recognize what major stress feels like for you.

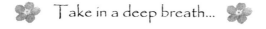 Take in a deep breath...

Caregiver Burnout

Sometimes the toll of being a caregiver is too much to bear. The last thing anybody wants to see is caregiver burnout. Below are some signs of caregiver stress that can lead to burnout. If you are experiencing any of these signs on a regular basis, ensure you are following some of the suggested self-care tips. As always, talk to your doctor if you feel your stress is adversely affecting your health and life; perhaps he or she may suggest other solutions based on your medical history. You may also want to inform your other family members so they are aware.

- **Physical Stress:** You might get headaches, have high blood pressure, even cry and feel sick to your stomach.

- **Sleep Issues:** You could toss and turn, get night sweats or have skin that feels clammy, feel wide-awake but exhausted, or just be unable to relax and rest.

- **Increased Sadness:** You might cry and feel a real lump in your throat, and think negative and sad thoughts.

- **Broken Concentration:** It might be hard for you to concentrate on the task at hand and even forget to do things you have planned.

- **Persistent Anxiety:** You may regularly feel inadequate or anxious about how you are measuring up as a caregiver. You may feel incapable of performing the heavy caregiving work required. This may make you feel angry or guilty.

- **Exhaustion:** You may notice a complete lack of energy and find daily tasks overwhelming.

- **Inability To Relax:** Does your mind not allow you to let go of your day? You might not be able to sit and just watch TV or chat with a friend. You are constantly thinking of the work that needs to be done.

- **Lowered Immunity:** You might get sick more often and for longer. Your immune system will be overrun by stress and unable to fight infections.

- **Extreme Irritability:** You may find yourself snapping at people around you, yelling orders, and becoming generally high strung and irritable. You may feel frustrated with an overwhelmed or helpless state of mind.

- **Increased Medication Use:** You may start taking drugs (even too many Tylenol or Advil), drinking too much alcohol, or smoking.

> **Helpful Hint:** Reminder - It is not recommended to go at it alone as a caregiver.

Regardless of how careful you are to incorporate self-care strategies, there are circumstances that can really take a toll on a caregiver, even though the tasks may not feel strenuous—including the length of time in the role. For example, if someone asked you to hold up a small tea light candle to help you light up the room for a few minutes, that would not cause you any issues. However, if someone asked you to hold up that same tea light for the entire day, then you would find it very uncomfortable for your arm and also for your back, neck, and head muscles.

What if you were asked to hold up a tea light candle for a few months or years? Certainly the little tea light you thought was easy to hold up in the first place has now become a health hazard for you. Compare this analogy to the role of caregiving. My hope is that you will be passing the tea light on a regular basis for others to hold to give yourself a break. For this to happen, you need to be open to asking and accepting the help.

Asking for Help

Asking for help is not always easy. It is a sad reality to realize there are many caregivers who don't ask for help when they really need it. Many people believe that asking for help is a sign of failure or incompetence. Tell me something; when a friend asks you for help with driving them to pick up their car at the garage, do you think to yourself, "This person is a failure?" Of course not! You may be thinking how pleased you are to help them out because if the tables were turned you would hope there would be someone to assist you. Isn't this what friendships are really all about? Recently, I met Wendy Yacboski, a Spiritual Life Coach and Ceremony Officiant, who gave a speech to caregivers that was very impactful. I asked her if I might share her message to the caregivers who will be reading this book. Here is what she kindly provided:

> *"Caring for others well contains an essential component that many of us were never taught about—that of RECEIVING. Perhaps you were taught that the desire or need to receive meant that you were weak or somehow inadequate for the job. If you have learned or perceived that giving does not require the self-care of receiving, I invite you to take another look at this very important area, for what we cannot receive, we cannot give.*
> *Receiving can be likened to the oil in the vehicle we drive. If we let it run out, we not only have a bumpy ride, the motor seizes! It is no different for us. We require the 'oil' of help from others and from ourselves, or our body, mind and spirit will seize! Replacing a vehicle's engine is very expensive. For us, the same analogy applies. If you are feeling 'empty' in your caregiving, ask yourself honestly, 'Am I allowing myself to ask for and receive help?' Just as your loved one needs to receive your giving, you need to receive from others who can give to you.*
> *Those who are good givers, tend not be good receivers; have you noticed? A variety of reasons could be at play here: a feeling of undeserving, a fear of inadequacy or rejection, or possibly a mistrust of the intimacy of receiving—for it is an exchange. None of these beliefs is the truth of you. To change any belief or habit requires practice. It requires that you be willing to receive and live a new way of being; to find out that it really can be different.*
> *If you find that you are not receiving, ask yourself, 'What is one small step I can take to help myself be open to receive today? A warm bath? A few moments of rejuvenating silence? A guided muscle relaxation exercise? Calling someone who understands?' Act on it; then ask yourself, 'How can I continue to take one receiving step at a time?' Put this into practice as regularly as you can.*
> *As you practice learning to receive, know that sometimes it will feel very uncomfortable, and perhaps even wrong, but this is just the old way of thinking. Your giving is a blessing, and so is your receiving. Step-by-step,*

Chapter One

open to receiving; build your openness to allowing others to give to you, too. Giving and receiving is not 'either/or' but 'and'. Like your car, you want to not only last a long time, but to have an enjoyable ride—regardless of the terrain you are driving through. While giving is demanding, receiving helps you to smooth each step of your journey."

The National Survey of Giving, Volunteering and Participating (2004) asked Canadians to choose from a list of reasons why they did not volunteer. There were many reasons including, "No one personally asked them." Think about this. Could it be that all you need to do is ask others for help? Once we change our mindset to recognize that asking for and receiving help is the best way to be proactive as a caregiver, then it becomes easier to seek the help we need and deserve. Asking for help takes practice for some people, and that is okay. Taking small steps at first to get the rhythm going may be what is required to feel more comfortable. With practice, asking for help will get easier. Sometimes having one or two items from your to-do list handled by someone else can make all the difference in the world. Hold on to that feeling and remind yourself the next time you feel overwhelmed how good it felt when you last asked for support and found people who were more than happy to help once you asked.

> **Helpful Hint:** Asking for help is not a sign of failure; it is actually the best way to be proactive.

Here is something else to consider; there may be people who want to help you but they may not know how. Perhaps giving them a specific task may be the solution to this disconnect. How about making a list of all tasks you need to accomplish in the next few weeks or months? Once this list of tasks is compiled, take a highlighter and highlight the tasks you could potentially have someone else do for you to lighten your load.

Now, think about the people in your circle of support who

have the ability in some way to assist you. List these people on paper in order to obtain a clear visual.

Here are a few examples:

- Your spouse (if the one cared for, perhaps your spouse may do one or two tasks, or parts of tasks?);
- Your children (don't shy away from those who live far away because there may be tasks that can be done from a distance);
- Your siblings;
- Your parents;
- Your extended family, such as nieces, nephews, aunts, uncles, cousins;
- Your friends;
- Your neighbours;
- Your local health authority or local government programs and services;
- Your church community;
- Your clubs or social networks;
- An accountant;
- Your local disease specific organizations.

What about private companies? For example, to give you a break, a home care company can match you with a home care worker who will assist you with some of your duties. These tasks may include cleaning, cooking, or assisting the person you are caring for with personal care. A home care worker may also provide companionship services such as taking your loved one for a walk, taking them shopping, taking them for a cup of coffee, or accompanying them to the local community care centre. Perhaps a live-in nanny may be more suitable to your situation? If finances are a concern for these paid services, make a note, but don't take these options off your list. At some point you may need to weigh the pros and cons surrounding private support and re-evaluate the value. In Canada, there are subsidized government supports

Chapter One

to assist family caregivers. Contact your doctor's office for the local contact information. Other financial supports may include Veteran Affairs Canada, not-for-profit organizations or even financial support from other family members. A helpful resource list can be found on my website: www.DementiaSolutions.ca

> **Helpful Hint:** Talk to your family doctor or local Alzheimer Society to find the appropriate supports in your community.

Self-Care

As the primary caregiver for your loved one with ADRD, you may be experiencing an array of emotions alongside physical symptoms such as those listed above. In addition, caregivers become prime candidates for depression due to the emotional stress and physical strain endured. There are a number of ways that you can preserve your health and reduce stress. The key to being an effective caregiver is to be aware of your stress levels and to continually build and maintain your own support team.

Although it may seem impossible to find the time, you need to take care of yourself first. As a family caregiver, if your health fails, you won't be of any assistance to anyone, including yourself.

To provide an analogy, consider the following: if you have ever been on an airplane, you may recall hearing the stewardess informing the passengers that in the event the breathing masks are lowered that you should be sure to place your mask on first before assisting others. The same rule needs to apply in caregiving. As a caregiver, your health is just as, if not more important than, the health of the person you are caring for. Therefore your needs must be considered first.

I frequently hear the line, "I have to do it all because there is no one else to do the caregiver work. Besides, I don't want to burden anyone else." I normally respond by saying, "I hear what you are saying, but tell me, who is going to take care of you when you burn yourself out?" This question certainly needs some pondering. It may turn out that the very people who you do not want to burden for some support in your caregiving role will then need to be fully involved in caring for you and your loved one.

Here are some ideas that a family or paid caregiver may utilize while taking care of themselves:

- **Inform yourself:** Learning about the disease or condition you are dealing with will provide you with insight, giving you a better idea of what to expect. Learn about caregiver burnout (by reading this book you are well on your way).

- **Be realistic about your abilities:** Being realistic about what you can and cannot do is important so that you are not too hard on yourself. Choose to accomplish what is most important to you and seek help with the rest. Learn how to delegate.

- **Remain positive:** It is not always easy but choosing to see the good (moments shared and abilities retained) instead of the more difficult moments will make caregiving significantly less stressful. As in all aspects of life, attitude is everything.

- **Find humour:** While this might seem impossible, try to find the humour in most situations. Laughing is some of the best medicine for the soul.

- **Seek assistance:** It is crucial that you obtain help with your caregiving tasks because caregiving should not be done alone. As a family caregiver, seek assistance with housekeeping, meals, or the personal caregiving tasks your loved one requires. For paid caregivers, seek support from peers or speak to your manager. Remember, asking for help does not mean that you are an inadequate caregiver!

Chapter One

- **Set aside "me" time:** Taking care of you is priority number one. As a family caregiver, you may not realize that you are entitled to coffee breaks. Make sure to set aside some time each day for yourself. It could be something as simple as putting your feet up and taking deep breaths, a brisk walk, or a hot bath. Make sure you are making time for friends. Social activities will help alleviate your sense of isolation and remind you that the world is bigger than your home.

 Time for taking in a dose of fresh air...

- Respite: Seek support from family, friends, or community to determine ways to allow yourself a break away or a few days off from your role. Recharging your batteries in this way is a good thing. A case manager from your local government support program could offer suggestions for community services such as a respite stay in a specialized home or adult day care centre. The case manager may be able to offer a reduced rate for these services, including home support from a home care worker or companion. Keep in mind that at any time a private home care company can be contacted directly to provide you with in-home support. You can find several of these companies in the yellow pages, on the Internet, or on my website's resource page.

- Share your feelings: It is critical that you share your feelings with someone you trust. This can be a friend, family member, support group, or a professional. Sharing will help others to understand what you're going through and could bring on new insights for you.

- Mind your health: Be certain to attend all your regular medical and dental check-up appointments and visit health professionals as regularly as you did before you began your caregiving duties. Be sure to have any new or unusual symptoms or problems checked immediately; remember to put yourself first!

- Plan ahead: Planning in advance for things like legal papers and final wishes has been known to reduce stress for families during a time of crisis. Making arrangements now may not be an easy thing to do, but certainly will be appreciated in the future.

> **Helpful Hint:** The key to being an effective caregiver is to be aware of your stress and build and maintain a strong support team.

Long Distance Caregiving

In today's world, people often have to relocate for work. Long distance caregiving for a loved one with ADRD presents its own set of unique challenges. Distance caregiving has been referred to as caring for a loved one from as little as a few miles away or from across an ocean—the range of the word distance can vary a great deal, depending on personal perceptions. Distance caregivers may be able to assist with managing appointments, paying bills, and other paperwork, at the beginning. As the disease progresses, distance caregiving may become increasingly difficult. There may come a time when complicated decisions need to be made. Perhaps your loved one has reached a stage in their disease where they need around-the-clock care and a decision has to be made whether they should move in with you (the long distance caregiver), with another relative, or into a care home.

If you are assisting with organizing supports from a distance, here are some suggestions you may want to consider:

- Seek out available resources in your loved one's community by using the Internet or contacting their family doctor.
- Remain in constant contact with siblings or relatives.

Chapter One

- When you are visiting, arrange a meeting with everyone involved in the care of your loved one and discuss options for care now and in the future.

- Arrange for daily monitoring by a friend, neighbour, or relative if the loved one lives alone. In addition, utilize any community services that are available, for example, a seniors' program that provides daily check-in telephone reassurance calls.

- It may be wise to inform neighbours of concerns regarding your loved one and offer them your phone number; they will need to know who to contact if your loved one is exhibiting strange behaviours. Organize support with various programs in the area such as Meals on Wheels, mobile hairdressing, transportation, homemakers, and adult day care. Many government programs have access to all these services and can point you in the right direction.

- As your loved one becomes increasingly forgetful, you may want to consider a program that can offer peace of mind, such as MedicAlert® Safely Home®. In Canada, The MedicAlert® Foundation and the Alzheimer's Society of Canada have partnered to create this new program. To learn more you can visit www.alzheimer.ca/en/Living-with-dementia/Day-to-day-living/Safety/Safely-Home. This program partners with all police departments across Canada to provide information to ensure the safe return of your loved one, should they become disoriented and lost. In the USA, the MedicAlert® + Alzheimer's Association Safe Return® is available. Visit the website to learn more: www.medicalert.org/products/everybody/package/medicalert-safe-return
- In other parts of the world, it would be best to contact Alzheimer's Disease International (ADI) by visiting their

website at www.alz.co.uk to assist you in locating your local Alzheimer's Association for more information on this type of service.

- If you are a long distance caregiver appointed as the Power of Attorney, you may consider automatic withdrawals for the regular recurring bills and prevent any potential confusion by stopping all bills from being sent to your loved one's home.

- Consider home monitoring systems; with technology evolving, there are systems available that provide added comfort and security for caregivers at a distance. Wireless sensors are placed throughout the home and can be programmed in a variety of ways to trigger alerts by email, calls, or text to any phone. For example: the system can be programmed to alert you, the caregiver, when the back door is open longer than five minutes or when the temperature in the kitchen goes over the maximum programmed temperature. Once an alert is given, the caregiver can take appropriate actions by alerting someone nearby to check in. One such company located in Canada is called Oceanview Safety and Security. To learn more contact 1 (250) 667-3839.

- Another type of technological device that I recently came across is called Claris Companion. Taken from their website, "Claris Companion combines the best features of a tablet computer, digital picture frame, mobile phone, and passive monitoring device into one elegant package designed specifically for elderly parents at home." To learn more about Claris Companion visit: www.clariscompanion.com

Let's address ways to provide assistance from afar if one of your relatives closer to the person with a dementia related dis-

Chapter One

ease has become the primary caregiver. Here are some suggestions as to how you may assist both individuals. It is important to remember that little things will add up to demonstrate your efforts to assist from a distance. Consider the following ideas:

- Inquire about the caregiver's health and self-care strategies

- Listen. They may just need someone to vent to without the desire to receive advice or assist with problem solving.

- Ask to receive copies of any medical reports to better understand and monitor the loved one's condition.

- Offer the primary caregiver time off by suggesting you trade places for a weekend or whenever you can spare time.

- Send a thank you card or a thinking of you card.

- Read up on the latest information on ADRD to stay informed and share with the primary caregiver.

- Consider attending a caregiver support group in your area to discover solutions for some of the problems the primary caregiver is experiencing. You may also choose to talk to a Dementia Consultant or Coach.

Changing Relationships

As the disease progresses, your relationship with your loved one will inevitably change. As you continue to adjust to your new role as a caregiver there may be times when you feel lost or confused. You may go through a period of mourning over the loss of your previous way of interacting and communicating. It is tremendously difficult to lose the emotional and physical closeness you are used to sharing with a loved one. If your feelings become overwhelming, make sure you obtain help by sharing your feelings.

If the individual diagnosed with ADRD is your spouse, your intimate relationship will also change. For example, your partner's sexual drive may be diminished due to the disease, physical illness, depression, or medication. Your sex drive may also lessen due to the demands of caregiving and changes in your partner's personality. This is common. There are other ways you will likely find to connect with one another. Again, a counselor will be able to support you with these emotional concerns.

You will also experience changes in your relationships with other family members and friends—who often withdraw because they are unaware of the disease and how to act and react toward you and your loved one. Explain what the person with ADRD is, and is not, capable of at any given point in time. As the disease progresses, offer ongoing information and updates about the disease to encourage your friends and relatives to remain engaged and involved.

Friends and relatives may refrain from visiting because they don't want to burden you by adding the stress of entertaining them. Let them know they're welcome to stop by, and offer ideas and activities that you could do together. Finally, you may be feeling like you have no time for others because of your duties as a caregiver. Let your friends and family members know that you still value your relationships with them. If you are feeling alone, and don't think others understand your situation, join a support group in person or online. This will help you find others in the same situation and you can share your experiences with them. You will quickly realize you are not alone.

Although caregiving can be challenging, it is important to appreciate the positive side—that caregiving can also have its rewards. It can give you a feeling of giving back to a loved one. It can also make you feel needed and can lead to a closer and stronger relationship with the person you are caring for. Many caregivers report they appreciate life more as a result of their

Chapter One

caregiving experience. Others have shared that being a caregiver has made them realize how much they can handle—to fully understand their strengths and capabilities—resulting in a good feeling about themselves and increased self-confidence.

Feeling good both mentally and physically is vital for anyone, including caregivers. The next chapter will be focusing on ways to maintain a healthy brain. There are many things we can do to fend off Alzheimer's disease and other related dementias!

Chapter 2

Proactive Ways to Maintain a Healthy Brain

"Do what you can, with what you have, where you are."
Theodore Roosevelt

Researchers across the world are racing towards a cure for Alzheimer's disease. As prevalence rates climb, the focus is turning to prevention strategies while the medical treatments continue to be explored.

According to the World Health Organization in a report released on April 12, 2012, nearly 35.6 million people worldwide live with dementia. This number is expected to double by 2030 (65.7 million) and more than triple by 2050 (115.4 million). Alzheimer's disease is the most common cause of dementia.

In order to come up with preventative measures one must first understand more about the brain and ADRD. Alzheimer's disease and many other dementias are known as neurodegenerative disorders. According to The EU Joint Programme: Neurodegenerative Disease Research (JPND), "Neurodegenerative disease is an umbrella term for a range of conditions which primarily affect the neurons in the human brain." What definitively causes this loss of structure or function of our neurons is still not known, and dementia continues to accelerate as a worldwide problem. What we can do is learn how we can build more neurons in our brain through what is known as Cognitive Reserve.

> **Helpful Hint:** It's never too early or too late to start boosting your brain reserves!

Cognitive Reserve

What is cognitive reserve and why do we need it? Dr. Sherrie All, Ph.D. from the Chicago Center for Cognitive Wellness best explains cognitive reserve:

> *"You can think of cognitive reserve as your brain's savings or retirement account. The bigger the balance, the more you have to cushion against losses that could really hurt you. By building up a larger cognitive reserve, you are saving your way to a better and more active retirement! Building up your brain's retirement account increases the chances that you will have a better quality of life during your golden years. This means that you will have more reserve left over to help you function day to day should you face any major deductions such as from a stroke or the changes that cause Alzheimer's. Having a large reserve can delay the onset of memory problems and functional declines, leading to greater independence and a better quality of life."*

According to Tori Deaux's blog post from August 4, 2009 titled "Why You Need a Cognitive Reserve (and how to build one), building cognitive reserve is like building access roads for the brain. The more brain cells and brain pathways, or roads that you grow in your brain throughout your life, the bigger your cognitive reserve account becomes. For example, the more streets you have in your brain the easier it is to get around between different parts of your brain, and the less likely you are to get stuck in a traffic jam or dead end when you come across an area of damaged neurons. By building cognitive reserves, our brain is better able to handle damage from injury or disease such as ADRD for a longer period of time.

Evidence is showing that the brains of seniors who were very mentally active throughout their lives had no obvious signs of declining cognitive functions. On the other hand, when the brains of these very mentally active seniors were examined after death, the results showed evidence of advanced neurodegeneration normally associated with ADRD. So, is it possible that cognitive reserves were built up by this group of mentally active seniors that allowed a wider variety of roads to be available in their brains?

In 2008, the Department of Neuroscience, Norwegian University of Science and Technology, released a study called "Risk-reducing effect of education in Alzheimer's disease" suggests that as we continue to explore the idea of building cognitive reserves, we may consider that higher education levels have a consistently protective effect on the risk of developing clinical Alzheimer's disease—according to a study released in 2008 by the Department of Neuroscience, Norwegian University of Science and Technology called "Risk-reducing effect of education in Alzheimer's disease." It makes logical sense that higher education will contribute to building cognitive reserves.

On 30 April 2013, the U.S. National Institutes of Health: National Library of Medicine offered evidence that cognitive reserves may be built up by lifelong exposure to multilingualism. The study called "Lifelong Exposure to Multilingualism: New Evidence to Support Cognitive Reserve Hypothesis" suggests that practicing multilingualism early in life and/or learning a new language at a fast pace provides protection to our brain that might be related to the enhancement of cognitive reserve and brain plasticity. As a result, it is theorized that any early or fast faced learning resultant of multilingualism heightens cognitive reserve and thereby protects and preserves brain functions from alterations during aging.

> **Helpful Hint:** Having a large cognitive reserve can delay the onset of memory problems and functional declines.

Exercising the Brain (Neuroplasticity)

Now that we know importance of building cognitive reserve through exposing our brain to higher education and lifelong learning, multilingualism, new ideas, and other challenging brain activities, it is now time to introduce the term neuroplasticity. Neuroplasticity is the scientific term used to describe the ability of the human brain to change as a result of our experiences. Historically, scientists believed that we were born with a finite number of brain cells. It is now known that this is not the case. Neuroplasticity tells us that we can exercise our brain to make our neural networks stronger and more flexible, just like we do with our muscles to make them stronger and more flexible.

According to Dr. Justin Davis who has a Ph.D. in neuromechanics and is the scientific director at nognz brain fitness in West Vancouver, British Columbia, "we have discovered that our brains are 'plastic' and 'malleable.' Our neurons are in a constant state of flux and form new connections with other neurons as we learn and develop new skills no matter what age we are." Our neurons can strengthen existing connections and even break connections. Neuroplasticity is what allows us to form the networks in our brain. We need these networks in order to process information, form memories, think critically, and make skilled movements.

> **Helpful Hint:** : Because of neuroplasticity, we can exercise our brains and learn and develop new skills no matter what age we are!

Brain Health

With certainty, new ideas on ways to maintain a healthy brain will be shared with the world as they arise. At present, the best way to reduce our risk of neuron damage through neurodegeneration is by leading a brain-healthy lifestyle.

While some factors are out of your control, such as your genes, many lifestyle choices can have dramatic results on your health and may be able to prevent dementia symptoms and slow down the process of deterioration.

Chapter Two

The following list is a compilation of proactive lifestyle choices and healthy living ideas paraphrased from several sources including Amanda Link's 29 May 2013 article on the website www.seniorsguideonline.com called "Having a Brain Healthy Lifestyle." Link's article originated from the work of authors Melinda Smith, MA; Melissa Wayne, MA; and Jeanne Segal, PhD, and it identifies the six key pillars of a brain-healthy lifestyle.

Six Key Pillars of a Brain Healthy Lifestyle

1. **Regular exercise:** It is critical to keep our hearts and lungs healthy and strong to pump all of the oxygen rich blood and nutrients to our brain. Any exercise done on a regular basis that gets the heart pumping and the blood flowing is beneficial. At least 30 minutes of aerobic exercise is valuable if done up to five times a week. Balance and coordination exercises such as yoga and tai chi could be done at regular intervals. Make sure your exercise routine also includes weight and resistance training. Consult your doctor to personalize a routine that works for you. Studies have shown that exercise results in improved performance on different cognitive tests as well as physiological changes in the structure of the brain.

2. **Healthy diet:** Eating a healthy diet is important for many reasons. Link's article states we should try to eat 4-6 smaller meals throughout the day and drink 2-4 cups of green tea daily to boost brain health. A diet rich in omega-3 fatty acids (commonly found in certain fish such as wild salmon, walnuts or other nuts, and even in flax seed oil), may also promote overall health and lower your risk of developing dementia by helping the brain to build and repair brain cells. It is important that we consume foods such as berries and dark coloured vegetables such as spinach and broccoli because they are a rich source of antioxidants that provide

protection from oxidative stress that damages our brain cells. We are also hearing lots in the news about eating a Mediterranean diet that includes meals rich in fish, nuts, whole grains, olive oil, and abundant fresh produce. Don't be shy to treat yourself to the occasional glass of red wine with your meal and even a square of dark chocolate to top it off. The nognz brain fitness website states, "Despite the fact our brains represent only ~2% of our total body weight, amazingly, our brain consumes ~20% of our daily energy intake! For this reason, it is essential that we start our day with a complete breakfast and make sure that [we] simply get enough food to eat each day to keep our brains functioning optimally."

3. **Quality sleep:** Your brain needs regular, restful sleep in order to function at optimum capacity, according to Amanda Link. Sleep deprivation not only leaves you cranky and tired, but impairs your ability to think, problem-solve, and process, store, and recall information. Deep, dreamy sleep is critical for memory formation and retention. The vast majority of adults need at least eight hours of sleep per night. Any less, and productivity and creativity suffers. Create a bedtime routine and maintain a sleep schedule. Take naps, but be smart about it. Napping for too long can make insomnia worse at night. If your brain won't turn off when you lie down, get up and try reading or relaxing in another room before returning to bed.

 Time to manage our stress; breathe in... and out.

4. **Stress management:** As mentioned in the previous chapter, the effects of stress on our bodies are wide-ranging. Chronic and severe stress can actually damage and kill brain cells in the hippocampus (the brain area responsible for memory), which ultimately shrinks the hippocampus

increasing your risk for Alzheimer's disease. Make sure to take time out each day to de-stress. This might include a walk in the park, meditation, a hot bath, or playing with your pet. Deep abdominal breathing as previously mentioned also quiets the body's stress response. Make sure to take a few minutes to breathe deeply every day.

> **Helpful Hint:** Deep abdominal breathing helps to reduce stress.

5. **An active social life:** The very act of being social is necessary to stimulate the brain, so get out there and have fun! Loneliness and social isolation are two of the most significant factors that put older adults at risk of suffering from ADRD. Our brains need to be stimulated through conversation, the sharing of ideas, and the company of others. It's time to join a group activity, take a class, volunteer, connect with family and friends (even electronically or over the phone), visit the local recreation centre, or make a weekly date with friends. If you have a partner, ensure you spend quality time together and go out regularly.

6. **Mental stimulation:** Exercising our brains with stimulating challenges may help us to think more efficiently, form new memories faster, remember old memories better, improve our motor skills and increase our mental endurance. With as little as five minutes a day of mental exercise, we may expect to see noticeable and lasting improvements in our mental performance.

We all understand the above is a very simplistic list and readers will immediately recognize that these six pillars of a brain-healthy lifestyle are common knowledge today. Yet, these six simple healthy living strategies provide a great outline for further study as readers seek ongoing ideas for living a brain-healthy lifestyle. Each one of the brain health categories contained in the six pillars have a multitude of researchers working on further studies with the goal of improving brain health.

At this point in the book, I would like to focus on the last of the above-listed six pillars, which is mental stimulation. It ties in with our earlier discussions of building up a cognitive reserve and encouraging neuroplasticity or exercising the brain for enhanced brain health.

To this end, I would like to present an excellent set of suggestions regarding exercising your brain to increase neuroplasticity provided by Dr. Justin Davis, PhD, who, as mentioned earlier, is the scientific director and also the product manager at nognz brain fitness. The following section on exercising all five regions of the brain is provided, with permission, from the nognz brain fitness website. According to Dr. Davis, we all need mental stimulation to push our mental boundaries and seek out novel activities and challenge our brain in ways it has never been challenged before. This may be done in a variety of ways, such as learning anything new, practicing memorization, playing strategy games, puzzles, and riddles. Your brain may also be challenged by trying something new, such as writing with your non-dominant hand or driving a different route.

Exercise the Whole Brain

In doing daily brain exercises, Dr. Davis recommends exercising the whole brain in all five regions of the brain:

1. Memory:
Here is how the nognz brain fitness website explains memory: "Memory is probably the easiest of the five cognitive domains to understand. Memory is the process through which new informa-

tion about our world is encoded, stored and later retrieved. Our ability to remember new facts and new ways of doing things is not only key to our ability to maintain independent lives, our memories are what individualizes each and every one of us. Our personal memories of past experiences and of family and friends are valuable treasures. Sadly, these treasures are often lost or become tarnished as we age and in tragic cases, with the onset of dementia. For this reason alone, it is necessary that we continue to exercise and activate the neural networks that form our memories. It is also important that we continue to find new strategies and tools to help us form new memories."

2. Focus:

Life today demands a lot of our attention. According to the nognz brain fitness website: "We live in a world of instant communication and sometimes the demands of work and family can become unbearable and seemingly never-ending. When we become mentally fatigued or over-burdened we can lose our ability to prioritize, our ability to identify important information and our ability to stay on task. At home, at the office and at school, we are constantly pulled in multiple directions at the same time and losing focus and concentration can result in us failing to meet our obligations."

3. Word Skills:

In terms of word skills, the nognz brain fitness website states: "Language is the highly evolved human skill that enables us to effectively communicate our thoughts and emotions with the rest of the world. Language is what allows us to grow as people, to share ideas with others and to form the social bonds that bring true value and meaning to our lives. And the fabulous fact about our word skills and capacity for language is that we can continue to improve these skills over the course of our lives."

Unfortunately, our abilities to communicate whether verbally or written can become compromised over time if we don't use them on a regular basis.

4. Coordination:

Referring to the nognz brain fitness website once again, it explains the importance of coordination as follows: "From the moment we wake up in the morning until we fall asleep at night, we humans are constantly on the move! And for most of us, our ability to make purposeful, timely and accurate movements is often taken for granted as we go about our day. But the truth is that our ability to perform the seemingly infinite number of goal directed movements we make is the result of our brain precisely detecting sensory information from the world around us and integrating it with our internal motivations to accurately execute the appropriate motor commands that tell our muscles how to move... Maybe it's not so simple after all? Unfortunately, as we age, this process becomes more difficult and moving about the world can become more challenging than it once was. For most of us, our senses tend to dull, our reaction times become a bit slower and seemingly simple motor tasks such as writing, driving our car and moving about to enjoy the things we love to do can become more difficult. For this reason, it is important that we not only exercise our muscles to maintain strength and flexibility to stay mobile, but that we also exercise the areas of our brain that are involved in coordinating our movements."

5. Critical Thinking:

Critical thought can also be referred to as our brain's executive function, according to the nognz brain fitness website. As such, "we can think of our critical thinking skills, as the analysis tools used by the CEO of our brain. Critical thinking skills are the tools we use to objectively analyze information, recognize patterns, follow logical rules, strategize, and solve problems. It is also the brain function that provides us with the ability to form the complex chronological and spatial plans we use to navigate our lives. Every day we use our critical thinking skills to objectively analyze the world we live [in] and thrive as individuals. Along with language, higher order critical thinking skills are what separate us humans from the rest of the Animal Kingdom. And anatomically speaking, the parts of our brain that allows us to think critically reside in the most highly evolved parts of our brain, the frontal and temporal lobes of the cortex. Sadly, it is most often our critical thinking skills that decline with age-related dementia. Our critical thinking skills also need to be fostered at an early age and throughout our lives in order for our brains to operate at their best."

To learn more about the five regions of the brain and unique fun types of brain games for each of the regions you can visit: www.nognz.com

> **Helpful Hint:** In as little as five minutes a day, we can have lasting improvements in our mental performance.

Hearing Loss and Brain Health

When exploring preventative options against dementia you may want to consider having your hearing checked. On 14 February 2011, the U.S. National Institutes of Health's National Library of Medicine published a study titled "Hearing Loss and Incident Dementia" by researchers Frank R. Lin, MD, PhD; E. Jeffrey Metter, MD; Richard J. O'Brien, MD, PhD; Susan M. Resnick, PhD; Alan B. Zonderman, PhD; and Luigi Ferrucci, MD, PhD.

The objective of this study was to determine if hearing loss was associated with incidents of dementia and Alzheimer's disease. The study included 639 men and women between the ages of 36 and 90, none of who had dementia at the start of the study in 1990. Cognitive and hearing tests were conducted over a four-year period, followed by patient tracking through to 2008 to monitor for signs of Alzheimer's disease or other related dementias. The researchers noted that of the 639 study participants, 125 were diagnosed with mild hearing loss, while another 53 had moderate loss, and six had severe loss.

Ultimately, 58 patients were diagnosed with dementia, of

which 37 had Alzheimer's disease. By cross-referencing their data, the researchers found that mild hearing loss was linked to a slight increase in dementia risk, but the risk increased noticeably among those with moderate and severe hearing loss. The "Hearing Loss and Incident Dementia" study, referenced above, concluded: "Hearing loss is independently associated with incident all-cause dementia. Whether hearing loss is a marker for early stage dementia or is actually a modifiable risk factor for dementia deserves further study."

When researching more on this topic, I came across an article called "Study Suggests Hearing Loss-Dementia Link" written by Alan Mozes and published in the HealthDay Reporter, which debated the results of the above noted "Hearing Loss and Incident Dementia" study. In this article, Dr. Richard B. Lipton, vice chair of neurology at Albert Einstein College of Medicine in New York City, was interviewed for his conclusions on the study results. He termed the study an "interesting" exploration that is predicated on "the widespread notion that chronological age may not be the best measure of biological age." He notes that although age is the most powerful risk factor for Alzheimer's disease, there are still many 90 year olds on the golf course. In other words, hearing loss may be an indicator that someone may not be aging well.

Dr. Richard B. Lipton, continuing to comment on the "Hearing Loss and Incident Dementia" study, as taken from the article written by Alan Mozes of the HealthDay Reporter, said "Another idea is that hearing loss might result from damage to nerve cells. That means damage to the hearing organ and inner ear structure called the cochlea, and the hair cells that pick up the pattern of vibration that the sound produces in the ear. And if there's damage to the neurons that mediate hearing, that may be a kind of marker for similar damage to nerve cells involved in memory and higher cognition."

A third possibility that may explain Dr. Lipton's interpretation of the "Hearing Loss and Incident Dementia" study results may be derived from significant evidence that hearing loss is socially isolating. If this was Dr. Lipton's rationale, then perhaps he is theorizing that social isolation contributes to the risk for Alzheimer's disease. As mentioned earlier, having an active social life is one of the ways to maintain good brain health.

As we continue our discussion of hearing loss and how it affects brain health, I would like to include another study in the debate. On 25 February 2013, the Jama Internal Medicine published another study by Dr. Lin and colleagues on hearing loss and dementia. Researchers looked at 1,984 older adults beginning in 1997-1998. Their findings reinforced those of the 2011 "Hearing Loss and Incident Dementia" study, but also discovered that individuals with hearing loss had a 30 to 40 percent faster decline rate in their thinking and memory abilities over a six-year period compared to people with normal hearing. The study concluded the following: "Hearing loss is independently associated with accelerated cognitive decline and incident cognitive impairment in community-dwelling older adults. Further studies are needed to investigate what the mechanistic basis of this association is and whether hearing rehabilitative interventions could affect cognitive decline." In other words, the above noted studies provide strong evidence to support the theory that higher levels of hearing loss may lead to higher levels of cognitive decline.

Our brain is amazing on its own, but it does require our help for optimal effectiveness. There are many safeguards we can construct in our daily lives to assist in maintaining good brain health. Several have been outlined in this chapter and readers are encouraged to pay attention to all the emerging information arising in brain health research. All healthy brain strategies are maximized when combined with a proper diet, sustainable exercise routines and stress reduction techniques that maintain good physical health. At every age, remaining focused on protective health habits and strategies appears to be the ultimate defence in preventing or delaying the onset of Alzheimer's disease or other related dementias.

 Time for taking in at least two deep breaths...

Chapter 3

Understanding Dementia and Alzheimer's Disease: What's the Difference?

"For myself I am an optimist—it does not seem to be much use being anything else."
Winston Churchill

With so many references interchangeably linking Alzheimer's disease to dementia, some people have the common misconception that dementia and Alzheimer's disease are one and the same. This chapter will assist readers to understand the difference. Be aware that resources available today to explain the term dementia do not provide one clear standard definition. Readers will be constantly challenged about these terms being used interchangeably, because authors find it challenging to keep them separate as well. Sometimes, unfortunately, you will have to be a bit of a detective to read between the lines and sort out the information most specific to the client or family member you are taking care of.

What really is Dementia?

At Personalized Dementia Solutions workshops, I usually start off educating participants with the question "What is dementia?" When faces lack confidence, I push the question further by asking, "Is dementia a disease?" It's interesting to me to see how some hands go up and others are slightly half way in the air. According to a 2012 report jointly put out by the World Health Organization and Alzheimer's Disease International called "Dementia: a public health priority," dementia is defined as the following:

> *"Dementia is a syndrome due to disease of the brain —usually of a chronic or progressive nature—in which there is disturbance of multiple higher cortical functions, including memory, thinking, orientation, comprehension, calculation, learning capacity, language, and judgement. Consciousness is not clouded. The impairments of cognitive function are commonly accompanied, and occasionally preceded, by deterioration in emotional control, social behaviour, or motivation. This syndrome occurs in a large number of conditions primarily or secondarily affecting the brain."*

So, if dementia is a syndrome, then what is the difference between a syndrome and a disease?

The Oxford Dictionary defines a syndrome as a group of symptoms, which consistently occur together, or a condition characterized by a set of associated symptoms. The same online dictionary defines a disease as a disorder of structure or function in a human, animal, or plant, especially one that produces specific symptoms or that affects a specific location and is not simply a direct result of physical injury. From my understanding, the syndrome (the cluster of symptoms) may suggest the possibility of an underlying disease or disorder.

I would like to share with you some other definitions of dementia from around the world. The Alzheimer Society of Canada states:

> *"Dementia is an umbrella term for a variety of brain disorders. Symptoms include loss of memory, judgment and reasoning, and changes in mood and behaviour. Brain function is affected enough to interfere with a person's ability to function at work, in relationships or in everyday activities. Several conditions produce symptoms similar to dementia. These can include depression, thyroid disease, infections or drug interactions. Early diagnosis is essential to make sure that people with these conditions get the right treatment. If the symptoms are caused by dementia, an early diagnosis will mean early access to support, information, and medication should it be available."*

Chapter Three

Here is the definition of dementia from the Alzheimer's Association (USA):

"Dementia is not a specific disease. It's an overall term that describes a wide range of symptoms associated with a decline in memory or other thinking skills severe enough to reduce a person's ability to perform everyday activities. Alzheimer's disease accounts for 60 to 80 percent of cases. Vascular dementia, which occurs after a stroke, is the second most common dementia type. But there are many other conditions that can cause symptoms of dementia, including some that are reversible, such as thyroid problems and vitamin deficiencies."

Alzheimer's Society (UK):

"The term 'dementia' describes a set of symptoms that include loss of memory, mood changes, and problems with communication and reasoning. There are many types of dementia. The most common are Alzheimer's disease and vascular dementia. Dementia is progressive, which means the symptoms will gradually get worse."

Alzheimer Society of Australia states:

"There are many different forms of dementia and each has its own causes. The most common types of dementia are; Alzheimer's disease, Vascular dementia, etc. There are a number of conditions that produce symptoms similar to dementia. These include some vitamin and hormone deficiencies, depression, medication clashes or overmedication, infections and brain tumours. It is essential that a medical diagnosis is obtained at an early stage when symptoms first appear to ensure that a person who has a treatable condition is diagnosed and treated correctly. If the symptoms are caused by dementia, an early diagnosis will mean early access to support, information, and medication should it be available."

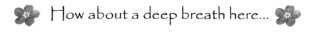 How about a deep breath here...

As you can see, resources available from these credible sources to explain the term dementia do not provide one clear standard definition. In my opinion, from reading the above, it is not straightforward whether dementia is a syndrome, or a set of symptoms, or an overall term, or a condition that has many types of dementias, or all of the above. In addition, the above descriptions raise questions for me as to whether it is valid to say "the syndrome of dementia (that has common symptoms), occurs in a large number of conditions" or rather "there are several types of dementia." Lastly, some definitions appear to conclude that dementia is non-reversible while other definitions appear to conclude that some types of dementia are reversible.

Dr. Robert Stern, Director of the Boston University Alzheimer's Disease Centre: Clinical Core gave a very effective analogy that has helped me to understand the term dementia by using the word fever in the Alzheimer's Reading Room blog on 14 May 2011:

> *"Fever refers to an elevated temperature, indicating that a person is sick. But it does not give any information about what is causing the sickness. In the same way, dementia means that there is something wrong with a person's brain, but it does not provide any information about what is causing the memory or cognitive difficulties. If these underlying problems of the dementia are identified and can be treated, then the dementia reverses and the person can return to normal functioning. However, most causes of dementia are not reversible. Rather, they are degenerative diseases of the brain that get worse over time. The most common cause of dementia is Alzheimer's disease, accounting for as many as 70-80% of all cases of dementia."*

Using the analogy of a fever is a very effective way to understand the term dementia because it is easy to relate to the many unknown reasons and conditions that may cause a fever in the same way that many unknown reasons and conditions may cause dementia.

Chapter Three

> **Helpful Hint:** You are not alone if you are feeling confused about the definition of dementia. Keep in mind, it is more important for caregivers to focus on understanding how to best provide care and how to best address the behaviours of someone diagnosed with dementia.

Changes in Terms Used in the Medical World

For those working in the healthcare field, changes in the terms commonly used when describing mild cognitive impairment (MCI) have occurred with the latest (fifth) edition of the Diagnostic and Statistical Manual of Mental Disorders (DSM V), which is the standard classification of mental disorders used by mental health professionals in the USA and Canada. MCI refers to having memory problems that are more pronounced than normal aging but not significant enough to be diagnosed as dementia. As of May 2013, DSM V contains the term Major and Mild Neurocognitive Disorder (NCD). This is just something else to keep a look out for in the near future when reading up on dementia.

Symptoms of Dementia

As more and more research becomes available on this topic perhaps we will be able to obtain a unified global understanding of all aspects of dementia. However, while the medical world determines the best definitions or terms for the various aspects of dementia related disease it is more important that we as caregivers concentrate on how we can best provide care and develop strategies to address the dementia related behaviours.

Armed with a somewhat better understanding of dementia, let's explore a little deeper some of the common symptoms of dementia: memory impairment, thinking impairment, poor judgement, personality changes, and communication difficulties.

- For a person to have memory impairment, they would have difficulty with recalling information that was provided to them only a short time earlier. In many cases, especially in the early stages of dementia, you may be asked "What are we doing for lunch today?" Sadly, you may have already answered this question three times in the past hour.

- For a person to present impairment in their thinking, you may notice a person having difficulty making change with cash or balancing their chequebook. When using a simple household appliance, such as a coffee machine or microwave you may see signs of difficulty in remembering how to turn them on, or set the dials.

- You may start to notice indications of faulty judgement. This may be expressed in the form of taking on an unmanageable task. A person, for example, may want to clean out all the shelves in the kitchen when they recently had a hip replacement and were told to rest for a few weeks. Or, contrary to their previous personality, an individual may start to say inappropriate things in public. You may experience a person saying out loud while pointing, "Look at that ugly purse on that woman!" while in earshot of the woman.

- It is common to start seeing changes in personality. These changes may include expressions of frustration, swearing, indications of passivity in a formerly assertive individual, refusing to go out with friends, frequent crying or outbursts, and becoming more dependent. The list can go on and on. Knowing the person will be more helpful in determining changes to their personality.

- Another common symptom of dementia is communication difficulties. An individual may start to use an incorrect

Chapter Three

word to explain something to you or perhaps may have increasing difficulty understanding what you are trying to tell them. You may notice changes in a person's writing abilities, some individuals may no longer be able to write a proper sentence or even remember how to write their own name.

When an individual is showing some or all of these common symptoms of dementia, it is best to have them reviewed as soon as possible by their doctor, who is trained to provide the formal diagnosis. The doctor will likely arrange for some tests, which may include blood work and a memory or cognitive test. Common cognitive tests at the moment include the MMSE (Mini-Mental Status Exam) or the MoCA (Montreal Cognitive Assessment). Once a formal diagnosis of dementia has been determined, it appears the next question should be, "What is causing the dementia?"

> **Helpful Hint:** If you don't already have a family physician, you may want to start your search in your province on the Federation of Medical Regulatory Authorities of Canada website: www.fmrac.ca/members/index.html

Overview of Some Common Causes of Dementia: Reversible/Treatable

There are several commonly known causes of dementia that are reversible and treatable. Another common term for reversible/treatable dementias is pseudo-dementias. In an article titled "Reversible Cognitive Disorder – Pseudodementia," an interesting passage states, "Estimates suggest that between 2% and 32% of older individuals who experience cognitive problems actually have pseudodementia...although pseudodementia is reversible, treating it can be as complex as treating 'regular dementia,' requiring a flexible approach and multiple treatment modalities (e.g., medication, psychotherapy, or a combination of both)."

The symptoms of dementia progresses and develops depending on the cause of the dementia. It can also depend on the overall health and circumstances of the individual. This means that the symptoms and experience of dementia can vary greatly from person to person. The sad news is that the irreversible dementias (such as the type associated with Alzheimer's disease) are the most common.

People affected by reversible/treatable (or pseudodementia) causes of dementia have options for treatment to function normally and symptom-free once again, provided they get their diagnosis early! The last thing you want is to be affected by a condition that can be reversed and not have it treated. This can result in permanent damage. Ideally, we need to put our stubbornness aside and seek medical attention to properly investigate what is going on.

According to the World Health Organization (WHO), lack of diagnosis is a major problem. Even in high-income countries, only one fifth to one half of cases of dementia are routinely recognized. Often, when a diagnosis is made by a doctor, it comes in the later stages, says Dr. Oleg Chestnov, Assistant Director-General, Noncommunicable Diseases and Mental Health at the WHO:

> *"We need to increase our capacity to detect dementia early and to provide the necessary health and social care. Health-care workers are often not adequately trained to recognize dementia. Much can be done to decrease the burden of dementia."*

As research on dementia expands, so too does the growing knowledge of risk factors and common treatable types of dementia. Below is a list of the most common treatable causes that have been summarized or paraphrased from a variety of sources to assist you with an overview.

Chapter Three

Depression:

Recent research is now indicating that depression in the elderly may be an early symptom of dementia. More specifically, having mild cognitive impairment (MCI) alongside depression doubled the risk of developing full-blown dementia, particularly when the depression goes untreated. Researchers from the University of Pittsburgh School of Medicine found that "Depressed older adults (defined as those over age 50) were more than twice as likely to develop vascular dementia and 65 percent more likely to develop Alzheimer's disease than similarly aged people who weren't depressed."

On 1 May 2013, the New York Times published an article about the research done by the University of Pittsburgh School of Medicine called "Does Depression Contribute to Dementia?" This article quotes Meryl Butters, an associate professor of psychiatry at the University of Pittsburgh School of Medicine and a co-author of the research paper saying, "We think depression is toxic to the brain, and if you're walking around with some mild brain damage, it will add to the degenerative process." The good news from this study is that full-blown dementia is less likely to occur if the individual obtains treatment for their depression.

Interestingly, there have been recent studies linked to gut bacteria on depression and anxiety. To provide an example, an article dated 23 May 2013 by Anne Angelone, MS (who is also a licensed Acupuncturist and Herbalist), titled, "The Link Between Gut Bacteria, Depression, Anxiety, and Weight Gain," states:

> *"Having plenty of beneficial bacteria, such as the Bifidobacteria strain, can promote production of serotonin, the "feel-good" chemical that prevents depression. Whereas having too much of the bad gut bacteria can promote depression and anxiety. This is because the gut is linked to the brain by the vagus nerve, a large nerve that sends messages back and forth between the brain and digestive system."*

Metabolic Dementia:

Metabolic dementia occurs due to a change in the body's metabolism. Some health conditions that can lead to metabolic dementia include diabetes, hypothyroidism, endocrine disorders such as Addison's or Cushing's disease, vitamin deficiencies (B1 and B12), cirrhosis of the liver and exposure to heavy metals such as lead, arsenic, or mercury. While metabolic dementia in itself is not treatable, often the underlying conditions causing the dementia are often treatable with medication. Another example is dehydration. Dehydration is very common and can present symptoms of dementia. Oftentimes, the individual may be unaware they have developed a metabolic disorder. If you suspect that one of these conditions could be a factor in the development of dementia, there are many tests a doctor can perform to verify your suspicions. For example, those who present a vitamin B12 deficiency often require monthly B12 shots to maintain appropriate levels in the body.

Delirium:

Delirium is a serious disturbance in a person's mental abilities that results in a decreased awareness of one's environment and confused thinking according to the Mayo Clinic. The onset of delirium is usually sudden, often within hours or a few days. Contributing factors that lead to delirium are: infection, surgery, chronic medical illness, medication, and drug or alcohol abuse. The symptoms of delirium and dementia can be similar therefore an accurate diagnosis is required. In the elderly, delirium is quite common.

   Dr. Daniel Davis of the University of Cambridge discovered that older people who experience episodes of delirium are far more likely to develop dementia at a later date. In fact, people who experienced delirium had an eight-fold risk in developing dementia. Dr. Davis notes, "Because some delirium

Chapter Three

is preventable, it is plausible that delirium prevention may lead to dementia prevention." As stated by Dr. Davis, some episodes of delirium are preventable, such as those from infections. The key is to ensure symptoms are monitored and treated early and appropriately.

Urinary Tract Infections (UTIs):

Urinary tract infections can cause a state of confusion, or delirium, in elderly individuals and worsen symptoms for those with dementia. UTIs occur more frequently in women than men and are more common in those requiring full-time care, using catheters, or wearing incontinence aids. For those without prior symptoms of dementia, the change in demeanor will be very sudden, often occurring within one to three days.

Jeffrey Kurz, author of the article "Doctor Raises Awareness of Link Between Dementia, Urinary Tract Infections," explains that the reason elderly people with UTIs experience delirium is due to the fact that older people have weaker blood vessel walls and vessels in the brain become more permeable, resulting in bacteria infecting the blood stream. Luckily, the test for UTI is a simple urine dip test. If symptoms of delirium or confusion rapidly occur, be sure to have a doctor test for a UTI. In order to prevent a UTI from occurring, ensure the individual drinks lots of fluids, eats foods high in fiber, gets plenty of exercise, practices good hygiene, avoids the use of talcum powder, and remind women to wipe front to back after using the toilet.

Other Infections:

Side effects of your body trying to fight off an infection, especially a fever, can result in dementia. According to the Division of Geriatric in S. John-Addolorata Hospital, in Rome, Italy, the most common infections that affect the brain with this effect include meningitis, encephalitis, Lyme disease, and syphilis. Conditions that compromise the immune system, such as leukemia and HIV/AIDS can also cause symptoms of dementia. Essentially, viruses, bacteria, and parasites destroy healthy brain cells resulting in dementia. Typically, this occurs in the later stages of severe infections. Inflammation is believed to play a pivotal role in dementia, but its role is still unclear.

Traumatic Brain Injury:

Traumatic brain injury (TBI) results from an impact to the head that disrupts normal brain function. TBI is a significant threat to cognitive health and can have long lasting or even permanent effects. According to the Alzheimer's Association, there are also certain types of TBI that may increase the risk of developing Alzheimer's disease or other forms of dementia years after the injury takes place. Possible causes for TBI include wounds that penetrate the skull and brain, serious falls, vehicle accidents, sports injuries, and concussions. Many TBIs are classified as mild because they're not life threatening. The severity of symptoms depends on whether the injury is mild, moderate, or severe. According to the Alzheimer's Association, the symptoms of a brain injury include unconsciousness, confusion and disorientation, headache, dizziness, blurry vision, nausea, and vomiting. In addition, the injury victim may not be able to remember the cause of the injury or the events that occurred immediately before or up to 24 hours after the injury.

Additional Causes of Reversible Dementia:

A few other causes of dementia that are treatable consist of poisoning, brain tumours, and heart and lung problems. Poisoning can include everything from heavy metal or carbon monoxide poisoning to alcohol poisoning and heavy drug use. Although extremely rare, brain tumours can result in cognitive impairment. Chronic heart or lung problems can limit the oxygen supply to the brain also resulting in dementia-like symptoms.

Chapter Three

Living a healthy lifestyle can help prevent many of these causes. Many of these treatable dementias listed in this section will benefit from a healthy diet, supplements, and exercise. Annual routine check-ups are also a great way to catch conditions at an early stage and help prevent the onset of other, more serious, complications. If not treated appropriately, these reversible/treatable dementias can progress to reduced brain function, which can be debilitating. Thus, the circle takes us back to prevention and also early diagnosis (Mayo Clinic staff).

Overview of Some Common Causes of Dementia:

> **Helpful Hint:** It can't be stressed enough to see a doctor sooner, rather than later, about concerns of memory loss and other symptoms that may suggest dementia because it may be something treatable.

Non-Reversible

Dementia is not a normal part of the aging process. Unfortunately and very sadly, some dementia symptoms are not currently reversible and are incurable. As mentioned, the most common cause of dementia is Alzheimer's disease, which we will be exploring in more detail in the next section. The following is only an overview of the common causes of non-reversible dementia paraphrased from a variety of sources.

Vascular Dementia (VaD):

The Alzheimer Society of Canada's website states that vascular dementia results from reduced blood flow to the brain after a stroke or a series of small brain strokes (mini strokes). Experts say vascular dementia is also common in people with hypertension and high blood pressure. This may be due to having a genetic disease, such as, endocarditis (inflammation of the endocardium) or amyloid angiopathy (blood or lymph disease). As a result, cells in the brain die, leading to the symptoms of dementia. VaD is the second leading cause of dementia, accounting for up to 20% of all cases.

VaD is also known as multi-infarct dementia, which produces common physical signs including weakness in the arms and legs, tremors, and walking with short shuffling steps. The dementia symptoms that occur are memory loss, confusion, slower thought processes, and mood change and irritability, and many sufferers wander at night. It's important to note that not all strokes cause dementia symptoms, but it is an occurrence for some individuals after having suffered a stroke (Alzheimer's Association).

Mixed Dementia:

When VaD and Alzheimer's disease occur at the same time, the diagnosis is labelled mixed dementia. Many experts believe mixed dementia is more common than previously thought and is becoming increasingly common with age. This belief is based on brain autopsies showing up to 45 percent of people with dementia have signs of both Alzheimer's disease and VaD, according to the Mayo Clinic Staff.

Parkinson's Disease:

Parkinson's disease is a disorder that affects nerve cells in the brain, mainly in the subcritical region of the brain. Neurons die or malfunction and don't create the chemical dopamine anymore, causing the person to lose muscle coordination. The resulting symptoms include trembling hands, arms, legs, jaw and face, stiff muscles and slow movement, and poor coordination and balance.

The website for the Parkinson Society states that the dementia symptoms that are common in those diagnosed with Parkinson's disease are impeded alertness, withdrawal and change of mood and personality, inability to problem solve, and getting stuck on one train of thought and not being able to overcome this. Some researchers suggest that at least 50% of people with Parkinson's disease have some mild cognitive impairment and according to

Chapter Three

the eMedicineHealth's website, "As many as 20% to 40% may have more severe symptoms of dementia."

Lewy Body Disease:

Lewy body disease is characterized by abnormal structures, called Lewy bodies that build up in different areas of the brain and cause degeneration and death of brain nerve cells. Here is a description of Lewy body dementia according to the Lewy Body Dementia Association Inc:

> *"Lewy body proteins are found in an area of the brain stem where they deplete the neurotransmitter dopamine, causing Parkinsonian symptoms. In Lewy body dementia, these abnormal proteins are diffuse throughout other areas of the brain, including the cerebral cortex. The brain chemical acetylcholine is depleted, causing disruption of perception, thinking and behaviour."*

Scientists believe that this disease is related to Alzheimer's disease and Parkinson's disease, because of their very similar symptoms. Lewy body disease usually affects the areas of the brain that involve thinking and movement. It accounts for 5-15% of all dementias according to the Alzheimer Society of Canada.

At present there is no known cause of Lewy body disease, and risk factors have not yet been identified. There currently is no evidence that it is an inherited disease. Symptoms of Lewy body disease include memory loss, confusion, trouble being alert, hallucinations, and problems with posture and movement.

FrontoTemporal Lobar Degeneration (FTLD):

Frontotemporal lobar dementia is an umbrella term for a group of rare disorders that primarily affect the frontal and temporal lobes of the brain. These lobe areas are associated with personality and behaviour and affect the person's ability to function. Researchers estimate that frontotemporal lobar dementia accounts for approximately two to five percent of all dementia cases.

The duration of FTLD varies. According to the National Institute of Neurological Disorders and Stroke, some patients decline rapidly over two to three years. In other instances, patients exhibit only minimal changes for an average of five to ten years after diagnosis. People with FTLD often exhibit socially inappropriate behaviours, and they may neglect their normal responsibilities.

Pick's Disease:

Pick's disease is a type of Frontotemporal lobar dementia (FTLD). In a brain affected with Pick's disease, nerve cells swell and become abnormal and die, and abnormal structures called Pick bodies are present in the neurons. Pick's disease runs in some families, but the cause for it is largely unknown. As with other Frontotemporal Lobar dementia symptoms, the affected person will have trouble with logic, thinking, language, concentration and judgement, he or she may act inappropriately socially, and his or her character may alter.

> **Helpful Hint:** Don't be shy to seek a second opinion or ask to be referred to a specialist.

Huntington's Disease:

Huntington's disease is a disease that is inherited, which causes degeneration of nerve cells in the brain (Mayo Clinic Staff). It affects a person's functional abilities and usually results in problems with movement and cognitive function. Personality changes are also common with Huntington's disease.

Alcohol Related Dementia:

Wernicke's Encephalopathy is a degenerative brain disorder caused by the lack of thiamine (vitamin B1). It may result from alcohol abuse, dietary deficiencies, eating disorders, or the effects of chemotherapy. Korsakoff's amnesic syndrome is a memory disorder that also results from a deficiency of thiamine. It is associated with alcoholism. The heart, vascular, and nervous system are involved, according to the Alzheimer's Association.

Although Wernicke's Encephalopathy and Korsakoff's may appear to be two different disorders, The Alzheimer Society of Canada informs us they are generally considered to be different stages of the same disorder, which is called Wernicke-Korsakoff syndrome. Wernicke's encephalopathy represents the acute phase of the disorder, and Korsakoff's amnesic syndrome represents the chronic phase. Common symptoms include memory impairment, learning impairment, problems with balance, and other mental functions. Yet, symptoms can vary from person to person.

HIV Aids:

Dementia can result from the human immunodeficiency virus that causes AIDS because the disease destroys the brain's white matter. The symptoms that occur from the deteriorated brain are impaired memory, apathy, concentration, and social withdrawal (Alzheimer's AU).

Creutzfeldt-Jacob disease (CJD):

CJD is a rare neurodegenerative disorder that rapidly progresses and is deadly. It is caused by infectious proteins called prions that can attack the brain, kill cells, and create gaps or holes in brain tissue. The Department of Human Health and Sciences Centre for Disease Control and Prevention in the USA claim the majority of cases of CJD (about 85%) occur as sporadic disease, a smaller proportion of patients (5-15%) develop CJD because of inherited mutations of the prion protein gene.

Chronic Traumatic Encephalopathy (CTE):

Recently news about CTE has been hitting the sports world. CTE is a progressive degenerative disease of the brain found in athletes (and others) with a history of repetitive brain trauma, including symptomatic concussions as well as asymptomatic sub concussive hits to the head, as defined by the Centre for the Study of Traumatic Encephalopathy. Symptoms of CTE include irritability, depression and cognitive problems; better tests and imaging scans are needed to improve the accuracy of diagnosis during the lifetime of an individual with CTE. Up to this point, those afflicted are mainly diagnosed after death.

 Time for taking in a great big breath...

What Is Alzheimer's Disease?
Know What You're Dealing With

Alzheimer's disease is the most common progressive, degenerative type of dementia, and it is not reversible. Continuous progress in the research and science surrounding the disease is encouraging, and every day more attention is being raised to inform and educate the general population; thus, a cure may ultimately be found. Nearly everyone is aware of Alzheimer's disease, but few actually know what the disease entails.

You may have heard of it referred to as the 'forgetting' disease or perhaps in medical terms as a neurological-degenerative disease. A person will likely be referred to visit a neurologist, at some point, when being diagnosed with Alzheimer's disease and many other doctors and specialists are likely to become involved in the diagnosis process.

It's a harsh reality to deal with because your loved one will gradually lose their ability to think, reason, and remember. Sadly, as this disease progresses to the later stages, daily support in carrying out regular everyday tasks, including bathing and

Chapter Three

toileting, becomes necessary. At the same time, due to the slow progression of Alzheimer's disease, it may be several years after diagnosis before this type of daily support is needed.

Now, please don't start to panic when you occasionally forget where you have placed your keys. We all do this! However, people with Alzheimer's disease will completely forget where they put their keys and often have much difficulty retracing their steps. They may even forget things such as where they were going while driving in their car and this forgetting does not simply last for a brief minute; rather, Alzheimer's may cause them to lose the ability to recall the memory of entire hours, or parts of days.

Keeping in mind that at the present time there is no cure for Alzheimer's disease, let's explore it in more depth. Please know that there are ways we can better understand people with this dementia related disease and to help them live a better life. In addition, there are ways that Alzheimer's disease sufferers can become more comfortable with our caregiving approaches through symptom and behaviour management.

As discussed in earlier chapters, there are many types of dementia syndromes that are attached to chronic medical conditions and diseases. Alzheimer's disease is the most common. In 2009, The Rising Tide Study: The Impact of Dementia on Canadian Society commissioned by the Alzheimer Society of Canada showed half a million Canadians had Alzheimer's disease or a related dementia. Of these Canadians, 71,000 were under the age of 65. That translates to 1 in 11 Canadians over the age of 65 living with Alzheimer's and related dementias.

According to a new study that was commissioned by the Alzheimer Society of Canada in 2012, "The number of Canadians living with cognitive impairment, including dementia, now stands at 747,000 and will double to 1.4 million by 2031. It is estimated that within a generation, the number of Canadians with Alzheimer's disease will more than double to over one million."

In most people with Alzheimer's disease, symptoms start to

appear after the age of 65, although there are those who develop symptoms before the age of 65 and this is known as early-onset dementia. Yet, recent research suggests that damage to the brain actually starts a decade or more before symptoms become apparent. More will be discussed about early-onset dementia in the Genetics section under the Risk Factors for Alzheimer's disease.

> **Helpful Hint:** Alzheimer dementia is not a normal part of aging. Early diagnosis is crucial.

Signs and Symptoms of Alzheimer's Disease

Alzheimer's disease affects everyone differently. Generally speaking, the disease results in an impairment of memory function, poor judgment, poor thinking, communication difficulties, and personality changes. Does this sound familiar? Yes, dementia syndrome symptoms are also many of the same symptoms as those in people diagnosed with Alzheimer's disease.

The Alzheimer Society of Canada has developed a list of the 10 warning signs to help individuals and families know what to look for. These warning signs have been summarized below:

1. **Memory loss that affects day-to-day function:** We all have moments when we forget names, or past activities and tasks that we promised we would do. A person with Alzheimer's disease may experience these memory laps on a more frequent basis and may begin to experience daily frustrations and challenges with their short-term memory.

2. **Difficulty performing familiar tasks:** Someone who always made the apple pie at Christmas may no longer be able to follow their family recipe due to Alzheimer's disease. In the later stages, this may also be true for a daily activity

such as making the morning coffee or putting together a sandwich.

3. **Problems with language:** It is not uncommon for a person to have difficulty finding the right word. A person with Alzheimer's disease, however, may forget simple words or may substitute words that do not make sense, resulting in communication difficulties for all parties.

4. **Disorientation of time and place:** We frequently read or hear media stories about a person with Alzheimer's disease who has gone missing. This is because the brain is no longer able to recognize familiar surroundings. Difficulties determining the time of day, for example, whether it is 9:00 in the morning or 9:00 in the evening, are also common with Alzheimer's disease.

5. **Poor or decreased judgment:** Poor judgment will be presented in many ways. For example, someone with Alzheimer's disease may try climbing a ladder to do a task even though only a few weeks earlier they had a physical injury such as a hip replacement. They may also say or do things that are not considered inappropriate in society such as making a negative remark to strangers. Decreased judgment may also include wearing slippers outside with snow on the ground.

6. **Problems with abstract thinking:** Difficulties making change at a retail store or balancing a chequebook may start to become noticeable when someone has problems with abstract thinking.

7. **Misplacing things:** It is easy for anyone to temporarily misplace things such as our keys or glasses. A person with

Alzheimer's disease may put things in inappropriate places such as placing keys in the sugar bowl.

8. **Changes in mood and behaviour:** It is not uncommon for someone with Alzheimer's disease to exhibit mood swings that appear to have no apparent reason or to display a mood that is not appropriate for the circumstance.

9. **Changes in personality:** Be mindful that a personality can change due to changes in the brain. Often I have heard, "Grandma used to be so sweet but now she is swearing like a trucker!" I have also heard, "Grandpa used to be grumpy when we visited, now he is so calm and happy all the time."

10. **Loss of initiative:** Not feeling in the mood to socialize or perform work around the house can happen to us all. However, a person with Alzheimer's disease may become very passive, and require someone to encourage them to get involved by providing gentle motivation or cues.

The brain tissue of an individual with Alzheimer's disease has many fewer nerve cells and synapses than a healthy brain. In advanced Alzheimer's disease, most of the cortex in the brain is seriously damaged because of this widespread cell death resulting in brain shrinkage (Alzheimer's Association). Scientists are not absolutely sure what causes cell death and tissue loss in the Alzheimer's brain, but the amyloid-beta plaques and tau protein/Neurofibrillary tangles are the prime suspects that we will be discussing in more detail under the section 'More In-Depth Information and Background on Alzheimer's Disease.'

Alzheimer's disease can also bring about erratic behaviour, increased agitation, mood fluctuations, difficulties performing familiar tasks, dependence on others, apathy, changes in their internal clock, increased sleepiness, and a loss of control over bodily functions. These symptoms can appear at any stage of the disease and vary in severity, but as the disease progresses, so do

Chapter Three

the symptoms. According to the explanations provided on Mayo Clinic's website regarding the stages of Alzheimer's disease, "On average, people live for 8 to 10 years after the initial diagnosis; but some may live longer and their symptoms will last for as long they live, even as long as 20 years".

> **Helpful Hint:** No two people progress through the stages of Alzheimer's disease in the same way.

As the disease progresses, most people with Alzheimer's disease require assistance with their daily needs including cleaning, changing, feeding, and toileting. Some individuals with Alzheimer's disease live at home with the help of a caregiver, while others live in long-term care homes. More often than not, the burden of care falls upon family and/or friends of the individual with Alzheimer's disease. As previously mentioned, this caregiver role can be tremendously challenging for all types of caregivers.

Sadly, family caregivers are compelled to watch the slow changes of the person they once knew and it is often very difficult to accept. It is hard to process the fact that their loved one will never revert back to being the person they once were. It is hurtful to accept that the previous emotional connections, such as providing you with advice about the grandchildren or your previous delight as they spoiled the grandchildren, are forever gone. Also, it is painful to realize that many of the activities and outings that you used to do together are no longer possible. It cannot be stressed enough that it is vitally important that family caregivers obtain help on this journey to avoid the dreadful and highly common caregiver burnout.

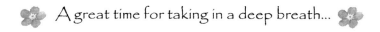
A great time for taking in a deep breath...

Stages of Alzheimer's Disease

Although everyone experiences Alzheimer's differently, symptoms normally progress in a series of stages. There are many different theories available to explain the stages of Alzheimer's disease; which have been described as ranging from three, four, five, or even to seven stages. In this book, we are going to concentrate on five stages.

To learn more about all the stages of Alzheimer's disease, please refer to the "Additional Resources" page found on my website at www.DementiaSolutions.ca.

According to the Mayo Clinic, a non-profit research and education organization, there are five stages associated with Alzheimer's disease: Preclinical Alzheimer's disease, mild cognitive impairment (MCI), mild dementia due to Alzheimer's, moderate dementia due to Alzheimer's, and severe dementia due to Alzheimer's. Although the course of the disease is not the same for everyone, symptoms appear to evolve within the same general stages. Familiarity with the general stages may assist you as you try to form an understanding about what to typically expect. However, it is important to realize that these stages are a rough guide based upon averages and generalizations. Several factors affect how long a person will live with Alzheimer's disease and at which rate they will advance through the stages. These factors include the person's age, sex, the presence of other health problems, and the severity of cognitive problems at diagnosis. Below are the stages paraphrased from the Mayo Clinic's website:

Stage 1: Preclinical Alzheimer's disease

Scientists believe that brain changes begin 10 to 20 years before Alzheimer's disease presents any symptoms. Because of this, scientists are keen to learn more about what happens in the brain during this hidden stage that sets a person on the path to developing Alzheimer's disease. New imaging technologies can now identify deposits of the amyloid beta proteins that have been associated with Alzheimer's disease. By knowing more about the early stages, scientists and researchers hope to be able to develop effective treatments and/or drugs that will slow or even halt the disease process before significant impairment occurs.

Stage 2: Mild cognitive impairment (MCI) due to Alzheimer's disease

Individuals diagnosed with mild cognitive impairment (MCI) have mild changes in their memory and thinking ability. At this stage, these changes aren't significant enough to affect work or relationships. It is common for individuals with MCI to have memory lapses regarding recent conversations, appointments, or events. People with MCI may also have trouble making decisions and difficulty correctly judging the number or sequence of steps needed to complete a task. It is important to note that not everyone with mild cognitive impairment has Alzheimer's disease. In some cases, MCI is due to a reversible dementia such as depression or a temporary medical complication. This is where proper diagnosing becomes very important.

Stage 3: Mild/Early Alzheimer's Disease (2-4 years)

This is the typical stage where friends, family, and medical professionals begin to notice significant issues with the individual's memory, thinking, and judgment. This is also the stage at which the disease is usually diagnosed. In the Mild to Early Alzheimer's disease stage, people may experience:

- **Memory loss:** difficulty recalling recent events and newly learned information or repeatedly asking the same question.
- **Problems with critical thinking:** planning a trip or birthday party may become entirely overwhelming. Lapses in judgment may result in unusual financial transactions.

- **Personality changes:** you may notice the individual becoming more withdrawn, irritable, or even angry. A limited attention span and reduced motivation are also common.
- **Communication difficulties:** struggling to find the right words and clearly convey ideas.
- **Losing items and themselves:** people with Alzheimer's disease commonly misplace things and will often get lost even in familiar places.

Stage 4: Moderate/Middle Alzheimer's Disease (2-10 years)

In the Moderate Alzheimer's stage, confusion and forgetfulness increase and individuals begin to require assistance with life's daily activities and self-care. People with Moderate Alzheimer's disease may experience the following:

- **An increased level of confusion:** individuals will tend to get lost more often and will become confused about everyday things, such as the day of the week. They need to be watched carefully as they may wander, searching for a place that feels 'right.' They may also take other peoples' belongings, as they tend not to recognize their own anymore. They begin to display confusion recognizing family members and close friends.
- **More memory loss:** memory loss extends to personal details such as remembering their address or phone number. Favourite stories get repeated. When favourite stories, or details of prior events cannot be remembered, new stories may then be created or altered.
- **Necessary assistance with daily life:** help with self-care activities such as bathing, grooming, and using the bathroom will be needed.
- **Noticeable personality changes:** increased suspicion of

others may begin to occur, the person may begin to see or hear things that aren't there, become agitated, violent, or experience sudden outbursts. Inappropriate sexual activity may also occur.

Stage 5: Severe/Late Alzheimer's Disease (1-3 + years)

In the Severe Alzheimer's stage, brain function continues to decay and physical capabilities decline. People with severe Alzheimer's disease generally have the following:

- **Communication breakdown:** communication is reduced to words and the occasional phrase, but it is incoherent.
- **Daily life support:** complete assistance is necessary with all daily life activities, including personal care. It is very important not to leave a person with Alzheimer's alone at this stage as they can inadvertently injure themselves or others.
- **Physical capabilities diminish:** everything from walking, feeding, toileting, and positioning themselves in bed. Towards the end of the disease, it is common for a person to lose the ability to swallow.

As Alzheimer's disease progresses, it is not unusual to think, for example, "My dad is a whole different person from the person he was before the disease." Alzheimer's disease changes the personality of an afflicted person—the way they think, feel, act, and understand. They no longer see or understand the world like you and I.

Sadly, this disease is a neurological disorder that ravages brain functions and processes as the brain cells are deteriorating. A good explanation of this process may be found in the book Still Alice written by Lisa Genova and published in 2007: "The well-being of a neuron depends on its ability to communicate with other neurons. Studies have shown that electrical and chemical stimulating from both a neuron's inputs and its targets support vital cellular processes. Neurons unable to connect effectively with other neurons atrophy. Useless, an abandoned neuron will die." As the abandoned neurons die the brain cells deteriorate and the physical capabilities diminish.

The "Memory Onion" Analogy

One of the most affected functions of the brain in people with Alzheimer's disease or other related dementias (ADRD) is memory. This is because the hippocampus region of the brain, which stores memory, is often the first region of the brain to deteriorate. The "memory onion" analogy has been very helpful to families and paid caregivers as they attempt to better understand the memory changes of those they are caring for.

> **Helpful Hint:** People with ADRD are better able to recall **feelings** than **facts**.

If you think about the many memories we gain as we grow up and live life, these memories might be referred to as resembling the layers of an onion. We gain experiences and knowledge, which we commit to mind in layers upon layers of memories. The outer layers of the onion represent our latest knowledge and memories, and as we get closer to the centre of the onion, we find our oldest memories and knowledge from our childhood. These memories are so deep-rooted that they lie resident in our brains as innate learning—take drinking out of a glass, for example. When you were young, you learned to drink water out of a glass and this knowledge has become second nature to you; therefore, it will be one of the later memories to fade away.

Someone who has ADRD can revert backwards through the layers of memory. In the latter stages of degenerative dementias; many individuals won't remember what they had for lunch ten minutes ago, but they will remember their school days as clear as if it was happening to them today. In fact, they're not only remembering, they are often re-living these memories in their mind.

I recall asking Harry who was in his 80s and in the middle stages of Alzheimer's disease dementia how old he was. He looked at me with a convincing face and said, "Well, I am your age of course." I was 26 at the time although many seniors thought I looked eighteen in those days. Knowing how old he thought he was helped me to understand where Harry was in his memory onion. It also clarified why he had not been able to previously recall having a wife and children. This was because this memory had not yet happened when he was in his late teens early twenties.

> **Helpful Hint:** People with ADRD may forget what you said, may forget what you did, and may even forget your name; however, they are more likely to recall how you made them feel.

Emotional Memory

Emotional memory is the memory of the feelings associated with an event, as opposed to the facts of the event according to the article, "Emotional Awareness and Emotional Memory" on the website of the Canadian Association of Occupational Therapist. Emotional memory is known to be preserved for people with ADRD. Knowing that feelings are stored rather than facts can help caregivers to ensure they are providing positive experiences to those they are caring for. For example, creating care routines with positive emotional associations may encourage the future cooperation of the person you are caring for with ADRD.

To help understand more about emotional memory in individuals with ADRD here is an overview of a study titled "Impact of emotion on memory: Controlled study of the influence of emotionally charged material on declarative memory in Alzheimer's disease." In this study these researchers demonstrated that a powerful emotional experience (The Kobe Earthquake also known as the Great Hanshin Earthquake took place on 17 January 1995 in Japan) reinforced memory retention in individuals with Alzheimer's disease.

Recall tests consisting of two short stories were administered to 34 individuals with Alzheimer's disease and 10 normal subjects. The two stories were identical except for one passage in each story: one passage in each story was emotionally charged (an arousing story) and the other (a neutral story) was not. This study showed that the arousing story was remembered better than the neutral story. The study's conclusion states the following: "The results provide further evidence that emotional arousal enhances declarative memory in patients with Alzheimer's disease, and give a clue to the management of people with dementia".

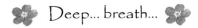

Deep... breath...

More In-Depth Information and Background on Alzheimer's Disease

The following section has been paraphrased from several excellent resources to provide you with additional information and background on Alzheimer's disease.

Dr. Aloysius "Alois" Alzheimer

In the publication The Discovery of Alzheimer's Disease, Hanns Hippius tells the history of Dr. Aloysius Alzheimer, a German psychiatrist and neuro-pathologist, identified the first case of pre-senile dementia, which we know now as Alzheimer's disease. In 1901, he became curious about a fifty-one year old patient in a Frankfurt Asylum named Auguste Deter, who was exhibiting signs of short-term memory loss and displaying strange behaviour. After this lady's death five years later, and with the permission of her family, Dr. Alzheimer did a brain autopsy and found extensive atrophy, particularly in the cortex. The cortex is the thin outer layer of grey matter in the brain that is responsible for memory, language, judgment, and thought.

Dr. Alzheimer then put silver salts on thin slices of Auguste's brain and examined them under the microscope. He found two types of abnormal deposits: one inside and one in between the nerve cells. These are currently referred to as amyloid plaques.

Dr. Alzheimer first presented his findings on Auguste Deter, at the 37th Annual Conference of German Psychiatrists in Tübingen, Germany in 1906, and then went on to publish articles regarding this and other cases. In another instance, the case of Johann F. was especially interesting to the doctor because the patient's symptoms included major memory problems along with language, movement, and other impairments, which started appearing when he was only fifty-four years of age. The autopsy of Johann F's brain revealed the presence of only one type of abnormal deposit: an external deposit (now termed neurofibrillary tangles).

The suggestion that Alzheimer's name is given to this syndrome came not from Alzheimer himself, but from his boss. Emil Kraepelin had recruited Alzheimer a few years earlier to work at his laboratory in Munich. Regarded by many as the founder of scientific psychiatry, Kraepelin included a description of the case of Auguste Deter in the eighth edition of his book Psychiatrie, published in 1910. By 1911, his description of the disease was being used by European physicians to diagnose patients in the US.

Types of Alzheimer's Disease

There are two main types of Alzheimer's disease: Familial Alzheimer's disease, also known as Familial Autosomal Dominant (FAD), and Sporadic Alzheimer's disease. It is important to note that both types of Alzheimer's are identical diseases.

With Familial Alzheimer's disease (FAD), it passes directly

from one generation to another. For example, if one parent has a mutated gene, each child has a fifty percent chance of inheriting it. The risk increases even more if both parents have the mutated gene. The presence of this gene means that the person will most likely develop Alzheimer's disease earlier in life ("early onset")— often in their forties or fifties. However, only five to ten percent of the Alzheimer population have FAD according to the TANZ Centre for Research in Neurodegenerative Diseases of the University of Toronto.

The majority of cases of Alzheimer's disease in people over the age of 65 are of the Sporadic ("late onset") form. It is still unclear as to exactly why these individuals are developing the disease. More information, again from the TANZ Centre for Research in Neurodegenerative Diseases of the University of Toronto, indicates that up to 68 percent of all cases do not have an APOE-4 allele, indicating that additional factors are involved in the late-onset form of the disease.

People who have the Sporadic form of Alzheimer's disease may or may not have a family history of it. On the other hand, if any relatives have had or currently have Alzheimer's disease, then a family member may possess a three times greater chance of developing it themselves. This is because some genetic factors shared by family members (aside from the inherited mutated gene that can cause FAD) can predispose someone to Sporadic Alzheimer's disease.

Risk Factors for Alzheimer's disease

Risk factors for Alzheimer's disease are still being studied. Some risk factors may be modified, for example, lowering one's blood pressure, cholesterol, and stress levels. Other modifications may be to incorporate brain and body exercises to manage obesity, as outlined in the previous chapter. Excessive alcohol consumption, cigarette smoking, and drug abuse are risk factors that may also have an impact, and may be modified with habit changes.

There are other factors that increase our risk of Alzheimer's

Chapter Three

disease and cannot be modified, for example, a person's age. Sadly, the top risk factor for Alzheimer's disease is age. According to the Alzheimer's Association in the USA, the likelihood of developing Alzheimer's disease doubles about every five years after age 65. After age 85, the risk reaches nearly 50 percent. Research is ongoing to determine why the risk of Alzheimer's disease increases dramatically as we age.

Genetics

Genetics is another major risk factor. We all have 22 pairs of chromosomes plus two X chromosomes (women) or an X and Y chromosome (men). Each chromosome contains thousands of genes like beads on a thread. We inherit genes from our parents that contain information and instructions that may be considered similar to blueprints for making who we are. These genes allow specific characteristics to manifest; for example, hair colour, height, or the tendency to develop certain conditions later in life that are passed from one generation to the next.

As more research is being conducted the Alzheimer's Association states that there is evidence that genetics play a role in Alzheimer's disease. Yet, having a close relative diagnosed with the disease does not exactly provide evidence of a genetic link. The good news is that only a small percentage of cases are associated with the specific genes that cause the inherited form of the disease (Familial Alzheimer's disease).

The most important gene discovered to date is the Apo lipoprotein E gene (APOE), which is found in chromosome 19. According to the Mayo Clinic, every person in the world carries two APOE genes (APOE types: 2, 3 and 4). These gene combinations are as follows: APOE 2, 2; APOE 3, 3; or APOE 4, 4; or a mixture of two types APOE 2, 3; APOE 2, 4; or APOE 3, 4. What they found is that people with at least one type of APOE 4 and especially those with two, such as APOE 4, 4, are at an increased risk of developing Alzheimer's disease earlier in life than those with the other types of APOE genes.

It was interesting to read on the Mayo Clinic's website that knowing whether or not you have the APOE 4 variant is not recommended because the results are difficult to interpret. This is because not all people with the APOE 4 variant will develop Alzheimer's disease. On the contrary, some people with no APOE 4 variant go on to develop Alzheimer's disease.

> **Helpful Hint:** Anyone considering genetic testing for Alzheimer's disease should consider counselling prior and following to the test.

As discussed earlier, Familial Alzheimer's disease (FAD) is not as prevalent yet occurs when a parent has a mutated gene that causes the FAD. Three genes have been identified, which if mutated in certain ways, will cause FAD. These are called presenilin 1 (chromosome 14), presenilin 2 (chromosome 1) and the amyloid precursor protein gene (APP) on chromosome 21.

Some other rare forms of dementia can also be inherited according to the Fight Alzheimer's Save Australia website. These include Huntington's disease and some forms of Frontotemporal Neurocognitive Disorders. These inherited conditions are very uncommon in the general population.

According to the Alzheimer Society of Canada's website at time of publishing this book, genetic testing for Alzheimer's disease is not widely available in Canada. It states that this type of testing is usually limited to people with a strong family history of the disease and who are enrolled in specific research studies. Some testing is also performed by referral from a family physician.

The website for the Alzheimer's Society in the UK states that there are currently no genetic tests that are sufficiently accurate for diagnosing Alzheimer's disease and suggests that anyone considering testing should also have proper genetic counselling. There are many aspects to consider prior to genetic testing. Let's consider some of the variables. For example, it may be important to consider how a positive genetic test for Alzheimer's disease may affect your eligibility for long-term care, disability, and life insurance. On the other hand, proof of a positive genetic test for Alzheimer's disease may be invaluable for a new couple that are making decisions about having children. Further, if a person knows that they are carrying a form of the early-onset genes, the Alzheimer's Society in the UK suggests it may be possible to take proactive steps to delay the potential onset of Alzheimer's disease. All in all, there are a myriad of factors and variables to consider when contemplating having genetic testing to attempt to expose your potential risk of developing Alzheimer's disease. Thus, it is crucial that genetic counselling is undertaken before any decisions to go ahead with testing are formalized. Attending genetic counselling will help you to fully understand the entire range of factors and variables that need to be considered. It is beyond the scope of this book to provide any comprehensive advice on genetic testing. Please seek genetic counselling if you are looking for guidance on this matter.

Other potential risk factors for developing Alzheimer's disease that are being researched include existing diseases or conditions such as hypertension, head injuries, diabetes, depression, hearing loss, and Downs Syndrome. Stress, levels of education, work history, and exposure to environmental substances or products are also being studied.

Current Research

Since Dr. Alzheimer's discovery over 100 years ago, there have been many scientific breakthroughs. In the 1960s, scientists discovered a link between cognitive decline and the number of plaques and tangles in the brain. A cluster of Amyloid proteins makes up amyloid plaques. Although the Amyloid protein is necessary for our immune systems, scientists recently discovered that the brains of individuals with Alzheimer's disease are full of amyloid plaques. As a result, one of the key areas of Alzheimer's research focuses on preventing the creation of these plaques by targeting the amyloid protein.

According to an online issue of the Archives of Neurology posted by the University of San Diego in April 2012, for an individual to be diagnosed with Alzheimer's disease, the presence of both amyloid-beta (a-beta) plaque deposits and elevated levels of an altered protein called p-tau (also known as Neurofibrillary tangles) is required. Interestingly, the study reports that in older individuals the presence of a-beta plague deposits alone was not associated with clinical decline. Anders M. Dale, PhD, professor of radiology, neurosciences, and psychiatry at UC San Diego and senior author of the study stated, "However, when p-tau was present in combination with a-beta, we saw significant clinical decline over three years."

Another avenue of research for scientists has been around the effects of oligomers in the understanding of Alzheimer's disease. These smaller, soluble oligomeric forms of tau have been associated with neuron loss and memory impairment. The summary of the 10 April 2013 journal article "The case for soluble Aβ oligomers as a drug target in Alzheimer's disease" in the Trends in Pharmacological Sciences states the following:

> *"Oligomer-targeting drugs should also confer long-term disease modification and slowing of disease progression, because they prevent the downstream signalling responsible for phospho-tau mediated cytoskeletal degeneration."*

In the study performed by scientists from the Icahn School of Medicine at Mount Sinai, in collaboration with researchers from the Icelandic Heart Association, discovered that a network of genes involved in an inflammatory response in the brain was a crucial mechanism causing late onset Alzheimer's disease. Their findings that were released on 25 April 2013 shows how inflammation plays a central role in Alzheimer's disease.

Valur Emilsson, PhD, Head of Systems Medicine at Icelandic Heart Association and also a senior author of the paper, was quoted as saying:

Chapter Three

"Currently, we see a long lag time between appearance of amyloid on brain scans of patients and the appearance of clinical symptoms. An individual's inflammatory response could well play a role in the disease progression, and an appropriate anti-inflammatory drug, given after amyloid is detected but before symptoms begin, could be an important part of dementia prevention."

Scientists across the world are regularly discovering new findings about Alzheimer's disease—it is exciting to read and hear about them. Hope continues. It seems something new is being brought forward to the public every day, which may cause some to feel bombarded. It may be difficult to weigh the pros and cons and evaluate the differences and usefulness between all the studies. Feel free to stay connected via the Personalized Dementia Solutions website or via Twitter to learn of the latest updates and research for Alzheimer's disease and related dementias.

Medications

At the time of writing this book, there are only a few medications available in Canada to help slow down the progression of Alzheimer's disease. Medicines called Cholinesterase Inhibitors are being widely prescribed. These types of drugs include the following:

- Donepezil: Brand name: Aricept (1997)
- Galantamine: Brand names: Nivalin, Razadyne, Razadyne ER, Reminyl, Lycoremine (2001)
- Rivastigmine: Brand name: Exelon (2000) Exelon also comes in a patch.

These medications help to increase both the level and duration of action of the neurotransmitter acetylcholine in the brain, which is the substance that conducts nerve impulses across synapses to cause muscles to move. Cholinesterase inhibitors also slow down the breakdown of acetylcholine and help brain cells work better. However, these medicines do not stop or reverse brain cell destruction and any loss of acetylcholine. The best these drugs can do is slow down the progression of Alzheimer's disease.

Another drug that has been gaining lots of attention and is being prescribed in tandem with one of the above Cholinesterase Inhibitors is:

- Memantine: Brand names: Axura, Akatinol, Namenda, Ebixa, Abixa, and Memox (2003)

Memantine is a glutamate pathway modifier. Glutamate is another chemical in the brain that is important for learning and memory. This drug is mainly used during the moderate to severe stages of Alzheimer's disease. Memantine claims it may provide benefits in thinking, daily functioning, and behaviour in people with moderate to severe Alzheimer's disease.

Keep in mind that all medications can have side effects and some of these can be very uncomfortable, such as nausea, vomiting, and diarrhoea. Some people may also be allergic or have organ deficiencies that would not allow them to take medications. These medications have worked very well for many but also do not work for everyone. It is best to consult a physician or pharmacist when discussing treatment options that should be personalized for your needs.

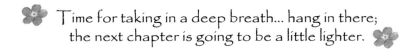
Time for taking in a deep breath... hang in there; the next chapter is going to be a little lighter.

Chapter 4
Behaviours and Coping Possibilities

"I have not failed. I've just found 10,000 ways that won't work."
Thomas A. Edison

As mentioned earlier, caring for someone with Alzheimer's disease and/or other related dementias (ADRD) is not always easy. Caregiving may be very rewarding, but when behaviour that is strange or difficult to handle comes into play, caregivers can benefit from some guidance. Your role as a family caregiver may need to be balanced with many other duties and commitments. It may be that you are required to deal with the stress of working full-time, while taking care of your children, and caring for your loved one with ADRD. There may never seem to be enough time in the day. As a paid caregiver, you may start to notice your client changing by becoming more agitated, or yelling at you, or saying things that hurt.

Behaviours are symptoms of many ADRDs and are not meant to deliberately upset you; it is a natural result of the damage occurring in the brain. These changed behaviours are often referred to as unwanted behaviours, challenging behaviours, difficult behaviours, responsive behaviours, or even disruptive behaviours. Whatever wording or language you prefer to use for these behaviours, these behaviours are not easy to deal with.

Before forming Personalized Dementia Solutions and while working in long-term care homes and with the Alzheimer's Society in Ontario, I came to realize many families had little understanding when it comes to handling these behaviours and often feel they have no other choice but to place their loved one into a care home. One of the goals of this book is to provide readers with resources that will help them to evaluate their own set of circumstances. Readers need a comprehensive amount of information in order to make an informed decision on how long the loved one, or client, should remain living at home, or in the community, and when it is necessary to consider moving the person with ADRD into a care home.

What is Behaviour?

The online Oxford English Dictionary defines behaviour as "the way in which an animal or person behaves in response to a particular situation or stimulus." In regards to behaviour in relation to ADRD, as the disease progresses there will be obvious changes in the person you are caring for. You may not notice how the thought processes change (decline); you will notice, however, that the outcome is strange behaviour. In addition, you will notice that situations, stimuli, and emotions can trigger adverse reactions, which therefore will emerge as negative effects.

Remember the analogy of the "Memory Onion" we discussed in Chapter three: if a person is firmly stuck in a past layer of their memory, could it be possible for increased anxiety or upset to develop if they are told they are wrong? Of course!

> **Helpful Hint:** Strange behaviours are common and a result of the damage occurring in the brain.

Possible Behaviours You May Experience

Here is a list of the most common behaviours provided by experienced ADRD caregivers at several of my workshops:

- Aggressive behaviour (physical/verbal)
- Agitation
- Anxious behaviour
- Delusions (false beliefs)
- Emotional fluctuations
- Forgetfulness
- Hallucinations (sensory perceptions not real)

Chapter Four

- Hoarding
- Hiding possessions
- Misperceptions
- Not wanting to bath, dress, or eat
- Paranoid behaviour
- Repetitive actions
- Resistance
- Repeating (same question over and over)
- Sundowning
- Wandering or pacing
- Wanting to "go home"

For readers who are not familiar with the above term sundowning, I wanted to provide a quick description. Sundowning is referred to as an increase in confusion around the time the sun goes down. During this time many of the above listed behaviours can occur or become more pronounced. It is thought that sundowning can be a problem for as many as 66 percent of people with Alzheimer's disease or other dementias. It is most common in middle stages of ADRD but can occur at any stage.

In this chapter you will find a list of possible coping strategies for addressing many of the changed behaviours mentioned above when they arise. Before we get to this list, let's first discuss the subject of conflict.

Conflict

Brenda Hooper is a Mediator, Conflict Resolution Specialist from Step by Step Mediation Services, a company in the lower mainland of British Columbia (www.StepByStepMediation.com). Brenda provides talks to family caregivers, where she speaks about the anatomy of a fight. She also provides participants with handouts that they may take away. She explains in great detail the process of how a fight can evolve. One of her handouts includes the following information:

The sequences of events in the retaliatory cycle are as follows:

1. **Triggering event:** Person A behaves either verbally or non-verbally that may be purely innocent or could be intended as hostile (a heavy sigh or rolling their eyes).

2. **Perception of threat:** Person B perceives the behaviour from Person A in a manner that Person B feels their self-interest is at risk. Person B may perceive "rolling eyes" as hostile or hearing deep sighs as Person A being impatient. This is the cognitive component of the cycle.

3. **Emotional Response:** People naturally and automatically respond to a perceived threat emotionally. Emotional Responses such as anger, sadness and frustration are used to protect oneself and is a healthy response. This is the emotional component of the retaliatory cycle.

4. **Acting Out:** Person B's emotional response creates an energy source and unless that energy is harnessed for collaborative problem solving, Person's B emotional response will transform into a behavioural response by acting out either with aggression or avoidance (or both).

5. **Repetition:** When Person B acts out either aggressively or by avoidance, this can be an intentional or unintentional event that can trigger Person A that there is a perceived threat. This sequence then becomes an endless loop from which there is no natural escape.

*Retaliatory Cycle adapted from Dr. Daniel Dana's book: "Managing Difference" –MTI Publications 2006.

Chapter Four

After reading the above information, it is not difficult to imagine how easily conflict can happen. Now substitute Person A for an individual with ADRD and Person B as the caregiver. With Person A having poor judgement, poor memory, poor thinking abilities, and difficulties with understanding communication, could you see how common conflict may surface for caregivers?

Coping Possibilities

Caring for someone with ADRD, who exhibits difficult behaviours as listed above, is certainly not an easy feat, especially if these behaviours are evident daily. Unfortunately, experiencing these behaviours is a common reality for many families and staff in care homes. In this next section, you may gain understanding, and perhaps put into action some of the listed coping possibilities. Please note: this is a list of possible strategies that have been used and continue to be used by many family and professional caregivers. Only you will know what will work best for your situation.

Take a break and come back later: Wouldn't you get tired of being told what to do all the time? So will your loved one. As much as you become worn out instructing your loved one, they may get tired of listening. Unfortunately, when you care for someone who isn't able to take care of themselves, you're forced to make decisions and take action for them. It may become necessary to remind them to do things all the time; for example, to brush their teeth, get dressed, eat their sandwich or watch where they're going.

One solution is to take a break and come back to the task later. Suppose you've asked your dad to get dressed for the day, and he has clearly said, "NO!" What might be the consequence if he doesn't get dressed immediately? This could be a great time to take a breathing break. He may me more amenable when you try him later.

Ask someone else to take over from you: When you care for someone on a daily basis, they become accustomed to you, including your tone of voice and mannerisms. This is both good and bad; it's good because it builds a mutually strong relationship based on familiarity and trust, but this closeness can also backfire sometimes. This same familiarity can become stale. If your loved one is too used to the way you handle their care, your usual caregiving style may not work sometimes. At times when your loved one feels confused, insecure, or weary, they may become extra stubborn and rebel against you because they are too familiar with your ways.

A fresh approach by someone else might break the spell. For example, it's the fifth day that you've tried to convince your mom to take a bath; you've tried to entice her with sweet smelling bubbles and a chocolate treat after the bath, but to no avail. Why not ask your husband or someone else she respects to step in? Perhaps with a change of person complimenting your mom and telling her how lovely she smelled the last time she took a bath, and explaining how wonderful it would be if they could share the treat after her bath, she might be more willing. When someone else tries, your loved one with ADRD might become curious about why the other person is asking and respond to their different mannerisms. This approach may take them off-guard and make them forget that they were being stubborn to you and not following your requests. In other words, someone else's request may seem like a new one altogether.

Accept these behaviours: Yes, it's easier said than done, yet, you need to make sure safety comes first. If the behaviour they're exhibiting is not hurting you, them, or others, you could simply decide to file the behaviour away as an acknowledgement of their new personality or their new little quirks.

When you come to the conclusion that a person's behaviour will not change, your attitude towards it should. If mom is constantly suspicious of someone taking her belongings, even if you give her what she thought she was missing, you know that she won't stop being suspicious.

Any phase or stage of ADRD may be short or it may last a few years. To accept changing behaviours is to keep responding appropriately to them, with compassion and understanding. For example, mom thinks someone is taking her keys all the time. You try to convince her she is wrong by looking for them with her and when you find them you show them to her and say, "See mom, no one is taking your keys, you just put them in your other coat pocket." No matter how much you try to convince your mom she is wrong to be suspicious of thieves, it may never work. It may be time to accept she is going to remain suspicious for a while and take the approach of kindly showing her where they are and then say with a smile, "Here they are!" and, "It's great that we found them!" No other convincing is necessary at this point in time.

Ignore the behaviours: I have witnessed this coping strategy on many occasions. I am not saying it is good or bad. Once again, this will depend on safety concerns. I fully understand how some behaviour can really cause upset for caregivers. The objective is to accept and not respond to the behaviour to see if it will stop. One example may be ignoring verbal aggressiveness. In order to ignore the person who just used foul language towards you, you need to acquire a Zen-like attitude, which will allow you to clear your mind of what they just said. Remember, it was not them speaking; it was actually the disease at work.

Another example could be every time the television is on your Dad taps his feet. You know he loves watching television daily, so it has become a constant occurrence in your home to hear this tap, tap, tap sound. Can you imagine the tap, tap, tap, of his feet? It can be very annoying! You have already tried asking him to stop to no avail. You know it won't help if you continually ask him to stop. You may sense that if you tried to hold his leg down he would most likely become upset with you. What you may be able to do is ignore this behaviour by leaving the room to do something else, or else you may want to turn up the TV so that the tapping noise gets integrated into the sounds coming from the TV. Some people may decide to use earplugs as a solution. The ability to ignore behaviour improves with time and exposure; your mind ultimately will try to deal with monotonous funny sounds and actions by eventually not taking any notice of them.

> **Helpful Hint:** Safety concerns should always be considered before any strange behaviours are ignored.

Involve dementia care professionals: The family physician, specialists, your case manager, representatives from your local Alzheimer Society, a professional caregiver from a home care company, and even a Dementia Consultant may be sought for support relating to the difficult behaviours. Experts in the field of ADRD will provide endless information, resources, and suggestions.

General information may also be found on the Internet. This material may range from how to get your elderly grandfather with dementia to stop resisting baths to what to do about your husband's early Alzheimer's detection and how to delay the disease symptoms as long as you can. There are countless studies, tips and stories out there on the Internet. Some places to look for the best helpful information on ADRD include the following:

The Alzheimer Society of Canada: (this site lists province-specific Alzheimer websites, which offer all the services available in each province and community): www.alzheimer.ca; or call Toll Free: 1-800-616-8816

- Alzheimer's Foundation for Caregiving in Canada: www.alzfdn.ca; or call Toll Free: 1-877-321-2594

- Alzheimer's Foundation of America: www.alzfdn.org; or call Toll Free: 1-866-232-8484

- The Alzheimer's Association (USA): www.alz.org; or call Toll Free 24/7: 1-800-272-3900

- Canadian Caregiver Coalition: www.ccc-ccan.ca

- Canadian Institute of Health Research: www.cihr-irsc.gc.ca/e/24936.html

- Alzheimer's Australia: www.fightdementia.org.au; or call Toll Free: 1-800-100-500

- Alzheimer's Disease International (ADI): www.alz.co.uk or call +44 20 79810880

- Personalized Dementia Solutions:www.DementiaSolutions.ca; or call 1-778-789-1496 for support from a Dementia Consultant.

Attend support groups: You are not alone, although I'm sure that's the way you may feel a lot of the time. Talking out the behaviours you are experiencing is a great way to cope. The best caregiving suggestions and insights often come from other family members who are on a similar journey. Besides the information exchange, a support group is a warm and welcoming place and an outlet for your thoughts and emotions around caregiving. The empathy, information, and encouragement that these groups can offer are amazing. You'll make good friends, talk about your difficulties together, and even gain contacts to call on if need be. To locate a local support group in your area, refer to the resources under the section above.

Educate yourself: There's nothing more daunting than not understanding what's happening to a person you are caring for and not knowing what you can do about it. You are doing a great thing by reading this book right now!

As mentioned earlier, there is an enormous amount of information about ADRD available on the Internet. One quick Google search and you'll be swamped! As a caregiver, you'll want to keep yourself updated about what to do at each stage of caregiving and the therapies that are available to help you on your journey. One great place to start is with the Alzheimer Societies and Associations as noted above.

The Personalized Dementia Solutions website regularly provides dementia related news updates in blog, and twitter feed (@Dementia__Help). In addition, our monthly newsletter offers true short stories of behaviours and creative ways to address them. We also have a section called, "Dear Dementia Consultant" where questions from caregivers are answered by a Dementia Consultant, which may be of great help to you. As well, the upcoming chapters in this book contain practical information on how to address behaviours.

For professional caregivers, it is important to stay relevant. Refreshers are also needed, because we can't expect to remember all we learned in a classroom setting. Sometimes hearing something again may trigger ideas about how to better assist your client. Speak to your managers regarding taking dementia training courses, or professional development courses being offered in your community. Cracking the Dementia Code™ is also a live workshop that can be presented to your co-workers. Contact us at: info@DementiaSolutions.ca for more details.

Give psychotropic/antipsychotic drugs: It is no secret we can be a drug-pushing society, and I'm not writing this book to preach for or against it. It is a choice that people make today, to give psychotropic drugs in the hope of softening the symptoms associated with dementia. It is noteworthy to remember that commonly known psychotropic medications, like Seroquel, Ativan, or Haldol, may have many unwanted side effects. These drugs need to be well prescribed and carefully monitored by health care professionals. These types of drugs are often extensively used in

Chapter Four

care facilities. In many instances, psychotropic drugs are referred to as a chemical restraint. If your loved one is taking any of these drugs it will be important to keep watch that these are well prescribed and monitored.

Psychotropic medications, often referred to as chemical restraints, are not necessarily helpful for all cases of dementia, but many people (family and professionals) feel helpless when someone with dementia is lashing out at them with verbal or physical abuse. The need to get these disruptive behaviours under control often leads the parties inclined to choose drugs as a possible coping strategy. An article in the New Hampshire News titled "The Battle Against 'Chemical Restraints' Inside Nursing Homes" mentions how geriatric psychiatrist Dr. Sandeep Sobti is working to lower the reliance on antipsychotic medications in New Hampshire nursing homes by pushing for alternative therapies to manage the behaviours. The opening line of the article states:

> *"Nursing homes around the country are under pressure from the Federal government to reduce their use of antipsychotics. This powerful class of prescription drug is meant for mental illnesses such as schizophrenia. But they are also being used on people with Alzheimer's disease at startling rates."*

The unfortunate reality is that the use of antipsychotic medications as chemical restraints for those affected by Alzheimer's disease living in care homes is not just a New Hampshire issue. Hospitals and care homes around the world are faced with this dilemma. Geriatric psychiatrist Dr. Sobti also is quoted in the New Hampshire News article as encouraging family to play an active role in treatment. He advises that family members should ask questions and carefully evaluate the answers received regarding the need for each medication.

> **Helpful Hint:** Certain drugs can pose a serious health risk for seniors and persons with ADRD.

Along with the "ethical questions of simply sedating" patients with ADRD, Alice Bonner with the Centers for Medicare and Medicaid Services was also quoted in the New Hampshire News article as saying that these types of drugs "pose a serious health risk" as they can "increase a senior's chance of falling, of stroke, and risk of death."

In 2004 a study titled, "Non-pharmacological Interventions in Dementia" published by The Royal College of Psychiatrists in their journal called Advances in Psychiatric Treatment, the following is quoted from the abstract:

> *"Pharmacological treatments for dementia should be used as a second-line approach and that non-pharmacological options should, in best practice, be pursued first."*

This publication suggests that providing drugs is a choice that needs careful consideration by the family doctor and pharmacist. In certain circumstances pharmacological treatments or psychotropic medications may be a needed coping strategy.

Often, when families do not fully understand dementia and how to address or cope with the resultant behaviours, it is common to experience significant frustration and stress. This added stress often leads to a major decision to find a care home for their loved one to move into. Now don't get me wrong, moving someone in the advanced stages of a dementia related disease into a care home is a very common occurrence and often becomes necessary for the safety of family members and caregivers who have become unable to cope in the home care environment. At the same time, I would like to clarify that my goal here is to ensure that everyone caring for a family member with ADRD understands that there are other creative solutions to help a loved one remain in their

Chapter Four

familiar environment for as long as possible and these creative solutions do not require excessive psychotropic medications to act as chemical restraints.

> **Helpful Hint:** Ideally, non-pharmacological coping strategies would be pursued first to prevent or divert difficult behaviours associated ADRD. The personality of the individual with ADRD along with their medical circumstance and the stage of their dementia will have major factors in the application of these possible coping strategies. There is no 'magic bullet' or one-size-fits-all solution to managing difficult behaviours and this fact underlines all suggestions provided in this book.

At this point, I would like to now introduce you to one more coping possibility, the one that makes this book more unique than many other self-help dementia books out there.

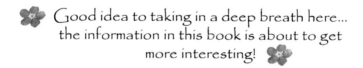

Good idea to taking in a deep breath here... the information in this book is about to get more interesting!

Chapter 5

The Dementia Code

"Not all of us can do great things. But we can do small things with great love."
Mother Teresa

For staff working in a care home, assisting individuals in later stages of Alzheimer's disease and/or other related dementias (ADRD) who are exhibiting concerning behaviours can make for a frustrating and energy draining shift. For family caregivers, being at a loss for ways to cope with the strange behaviours may result in the dreaded caregiver burnout. But then again, there is one other solution that can also be a coping possibility:

You can manage the behaviour!

Let's first understand more about the word manage. The online dictionary www.dictionary.reference.com defines the word manage this way:

- To bring about or succeed in accomplishing, sometimes despite difficulty or hardship.
- To dominate or influence (a person) by tact, flattery, or artifice.

It is the second bullet of the definition for manage that I would like us to explore a little deeper.

> **Helpful Hint:** Managing behaviour will need to depend on the individual you are caring for, their abilities, the stage of their illness, the kind of day they are having and/or the time of day.

Manage With Tact, Flattery, and Artifice

This is a touchy subject, but such an important one to address. In our society, many view tact and flattery as positive values, and artifice as a negative one; as good people, we always try to be truthful and agreeable. However, when it comes to dealing with later stages of ADRD, a condition that destroys a person's ability to understand social values and reality as we know it, we need to think differently and handle these special individuals differently. Of course we know that no two people with ADRD are the same and, as is written in the Helpful Hint box above, the success of using this coping strategy will depend on the individual you are caring for, the kind of day they are having, and the time of day.

I'm not suggesting in any way for a caregiver to be deceitful with bad intentions; on the contrary, I'm suggesting for caregivers to consider their loved one's or client's reality (recall the "memory onion" analogy); a reality that's alternate from ours, such as he or she may believe they still live with their parents in the same house as they did when they were younger. We need to have caring intentions relating to the person with ADRD at their level of thinking and the understanding to create more harmonious relations.

> **Helpful Hint:** As dementia caregivers, we need to change our ways. We cannot expect a person with ADRD to change their ways.

Managing behaviours of those in later stages of ADRD needs to come from a place of caring. Ultimately, you want the person who you are caring for to continue to feel somewhat in control for as long as possible. Put yourself in their shoes for a moment to visualize how it would feel to have someone take away your independence and control. When a person who has been diagnosed with ADRD is unaware they are making many unwise choices, but are fully aware of when someone is taking control from them, resistance can happen. This is one example of where managing behaviour can support you. Here is a more detailed look into the terms: tact, flattery, and artifice.

Tact: We use diplomacy, skill, and sensitivity every day, at work, in business, with our young children, and even at a family reunion with Uncle Jack who has had too much to drink. Why? It works well to ease minds and gets the message across without an uncomfortable hiccup or ruffled feathers.

Tact involves keeping the peace. It also involves delicacy and skill. Tact can be used in dealing with someone in the later stages of ADRD, by doing or not doing things in order to keep the peace. For example, ignoring odd or rude statements so not to create even more of an upsetting situation for everyone is using tact. You are doing this in order to keep the peace and you are doing so in a skilful way to manage the behaviour.

Flattery: Sweet talk, adulation, and praise are wonderful ways of flattering someone to make them feel good. We also use flattery on a daily basis—at work, in public, at a class reunion, even at a restaurant when we want to get great service. Who doesn't like nice compliments to make them feel good about themselves?

Using flattery in dealing with someone with ADRD in later stages works in a similar way: to make them feel good. By being friendly and pleasant towards them you are encouraging them towards obtaining or maintaining a great mood. Offering compliments may result in a feeling of appreciation and this positive feeling may go a long way in the day of a person with ADRD. There is an old saying, "Do unto others as you would have them do to you." Sound familiar? An interesting realization is that many individuals affected in the later stages of ADRD will have unstable emotions. Often it can be only a slight stimulus that can set them off into a negative or bad mood. This also can happen in reverse. A sudden smile or compliment can quickly set them off into a great mood!

I know this is not always easy to do; for example, perhaps you may feel that the person you are caring for does not deserve kindness for all the terrible things they may have said or did to you in the past. If reducing their aggression and getting them to cooperate is your main goal, then perhaps by saying or doing what you can to get them in a good mood may make your caregiving role and tasks more manageable. I will leave that to you to ponder.

Artifice: We were always taught that ploys, tricks, and lies are not good behaviour. This is because people who act in this manner usually have bad intentions. However, what if you have good intentions? For example, what if you trick your child into believing there is no chocolate left in the house, when you know they've had enough chocolate for the day? Or, what if you tell a white lie to your sister by telling her it looks like she is losing weight since she has been going to the gym just to encourage her to continue going? Or, what if you set up a tactic to fool your friend in order for her not to find out what you've planned for her as a surprise birthday party? Yes, we all tell these little white lies without a deceitful thought in our heads just to make sure a situation goes well or to make others happy.

Using artifice in dealing with someone who is in later stages of ADRD may consist of hiding things they shouldn't have, such as objects that are not safe. Further, using artifice may include saying things that will make the person feel content, at ease, and even good about themselves. Creating a guise to gain their trust and to convince them of an idea that will benefit them can be a helpful way to manage the behaviour and create a more harmonious situation. Of course the goal would be to not have to use artifice as an approach to managing behaviours in the first place, however when the truth is only causing more concern or upset for the one you are caring for with later stages of ADRD, then perhaps you may find artifice to be your best option.

Chapter Five

> **Helpful Hint:** Using artifice in dementia care is only used with good intentions when the truth cannot be comprehended, not used to cause harm.

Why Manage Behaviours?

Managing behaviours by using some or a combination of the ideas above works! Yet, I have heard several excuses and reasons why family caregivers, as well as professional caregivers, feel they cannot manage behaviours. These include having little patience, not enough time, being too tired, not having enough energy, and not feeling comfortable with it. There is also often a fear of the eruption of physical violence when trying to manage someone who is not rational or cooperative.

These are understandable reasons, but let me help you understand that it doesn't have to be as difficult as you may think it is. In some cases, managing behaviour can literally take seconds! Often when I hear these complaints, it appears to me that these individuals are not aware of one major important fact—

the Dementia Code

 It's time for a little stretch break! While you are at it, why not take in a deep breath...

It is now time to start you on the process on how to Cracking the Dementia Code! Before we begin, I want to mention that this next information needs to be shared with everyone who is caring for someone in later stages of ADRD. You may often find this same message implied in many of the literatures about dementia but it is not emphasized to the extent it should be! This message needs to be loud and clear and flashing like a neon light for all to see and take notice.

This is the moment you have been waiting for: the secret for Cracking the Dementia Code—for managing challenging behaviours is—

> **REALIZING ALL BEHAVIOUR HAS MEANING**

In other words, this means there is a reason for why the challenging or difficult behaviour is happening. If you truly adopt this way of thinking then you will be able to better manage the behaviour. As a result, this mindset will allow you and your loved one or client with ADRD to have a more harmonious relationship with minimal stress for both of you.

In 2010, WorksafeBC created a publication called, Dementia: Understanding Risks and Preventing Violence, which teaches front line care staff ways to prevent or minimize the risk of injuries resulting from providing care to those with dementia. Their book explains how when basic needs are not met, a person with later stages of ADRD can become frustrated, which may then cause behaviours to escalate. In my experience, unmet needs are often the reason for the behaviours. Unmet needs could be anything from being hunger, thirst, needing to use a toilet, not feeling listened to, not feeling safe, not knowing important information such as where they live, needing reassurance of any kind, and the list goes on.

How to Crack the Dementia Code

In these last two chapters, we discussed the coping possibilities to help you deal with the behaviours of ADRD including manage the behaviours. However, in order to manage the behaviours we need to understand why the behaviour is happening in the first place, such as determining the unmet need.

Chapter Five

Dr. Sobti, the doctor mentioned in chapter four regarding concern for the overuse of psychotropic drugs, in the article Battle Against 'Chemical Restraints' Inside Nursing Homes, is urging more patience among staff and more focus on what is causing the behaviours. He is suggesting concentrating on alternatives to using medicine to calm someone down. It sounds simple, but he says "caregivers don't get the needed training for behavioural issues." The next few chapters are designed to assist you the caregiver with obtaining a new way of thinking and a new pathway for managing behavioural issues.

We know that people in the later stages of ADRD will not always think critically, understand meaning or what's really going on in a situation. This will depend on the individual you are caring for such as their abilities, their medical condition, the stage they are in, the kind of day they are having, and the time of day. We also know that those in later stages of ADRD will have difficulty expressing themselves emotionally and verbally, so how can their behaviour have meaning?

The "Memory Onion" Analogy comes in handy here. Those in later stages of ADRD retain their natural instincts, coupled with what they learned in the past years. It is common to observe them reverting back to these older memories when their most recent memories begin to deteriorate. The emotions that result from the older memories may be illogical and even heightened. It will be apparent that they exist in a reality that is alternate to ours.

Concurrently, it will be obvious that they are feeling and reacting to this alternative reality. For the most part, other than in the final stage of ADRD, they will be able to innately understand their own needs in the most basic sense. This means they may feel pain, fear, anger, happiness, tiredness, and just about any other basic human feeling. However, they may not be able to communicate this well or express themselves in a way that is considered normal in our culture.

Now that we understand that all behaviour has meaning, the next step is to figure out why the behaviour is happening—it

Hint: All behaviour has meaning.

Asking "Why?"

When you ask yourself the question "why," it actually sets in motion the critical thinking part of your brain. According to the Alberta Education website, critical thinking is reflective thinking focused on deciding what would be sensible or reasonable to believe or do in a given situation. What better way to spark this natural reflective thinking than to ask yourself a question, "why?"

The Power of Why is a book written by Amanda Lang, a CBC journalist from Canada and it was published in 2012. In this book she explains how asking the right questions has changed the world and discusses how asking "why" can change you. The publisher, Harper Collins has the following book description on their website:

> *"Instead of obsessing over working 'smarter,' we ought to focus on the instinctive urge to question that's so natural for young children. As Lang shows, it's possible to reignite that instinct at any age and to become more innovative and productive—as well as more fulfilled in our jobs and happier in our relationships. That's the power of why."*

Amanda Lang writes the following verse in her book, Want to change your life? Start asking yourself "why" not "how" questions.

After reading this amazing quotation, it was no surprise when my brain automatically wanted to relate to the work that is being done by so many in the world of dementia care.
Therefore:

Chapter Five

"Want to better manage the difficult behaviours of someone with dementia? Start by asking yourself "why" not "how" questions.
Karen Tyrell, CDP, CPCA

It is interesting how many people who are struggling to care for someone with ADRD will often ask me "how" questions. For example, "How do we get my grandmother to stop pulling off the bed sheets?" or "How do I stop my dad from asking every day when the next meal is coming?" By asking questions such as why your grandmother is pulling all the bed sheets off of the bed, or why your dad is asking for her next meal, you are beginning the process of cracking the dementia code. After asking yourself the initial question of why, it is now time to put on your detective hat to determine this answer in order to come up with the appropriate solution(s). By jumping to the "how do we solve" mode, rather than the "why is the behaviour happening" mode, you could be wasting your time and energy. The goal here is to come up with effective solutions for your situation. You may be missing the opportunity to discover the real reason why and the solutions that will make the difference for you.

> **Helpful Hint:** Those in later stages of ADRD are often not knowingly in an alternative reality. It is the disease at work.

Chapter 6
Gathering the Ph.A.C.T.S.™

"There is no exercise better for the heart than reaching down and lifting people up."
John Holmes

As any good mystery detective, you must gather your facts, or in the case of cracking the dementia code, you need to gather the Ph.A.C.T.S™:

Ph: Physical
A: Ask them
C: Consider Cognitive Concerns
T: Triggers
S: Scan the Environment

Becoming a Detective

Once you have asked yourself why and put on your imaginary detective hat, your brain is now ready to examine the Ph.A.C.T.S.™, and to investigate why the behaviour is happening.

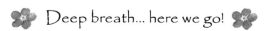
Deep breath... here we go!

Ph stands for Physical: Is something physical happening to account for why the person is exhibiting strange behaviour? Often behaviours are a result of pain. What is happening that may be prompting them to act out in various inappropriate ways? Is grandma expressing anger each time she is assisted to take a bath, because the water is too hot? Does she kick you when you are trying to put on a shoe on her sore foot? Is your wife prone to constipation? Could this be why she is crying? Could it be pain related to arthritis or diabetes? Look at what could be going on with the body by way of visually watching for facial clues and expressions or by listening carefully for sounds, such as groans. These are only a few examples. There are hundreds of others. Be a detective to determine if physical issues are a factor in the behaviour you are witnessing.

For example, many people in later stages of ADRD, do not get enough fluid because they no longer recognize the sensation of thirst and may forget to drink. They also may forget how to drink or how to prepare a drink, which is common in the later stages. All caregivers should understand symptoms of dehydration. They may include confusion, dizziness, skin that appears dry, flushing, fever, and rapid pulse. Some examples of other physical issues that may cause unusual behaviours include the following:

- Hunger, as well as thirst/dehydration (detailed above)
- Fatigue
- Sleep deprivation or disruption
- Discomfort
- Acute illness
- Chronic pain/illness
- Depression
- An underlying psychiatric illness
- Physical changes in the brain/body
- Adverse side effects of their medications
- Over medicated or under medicated
- Impaired vision or hearing

Helpful Hint: Acute illnesses such as a Urinary Tract Infection, Bladder Infection, or an Upper Respiratory Infection such as the flu or pneumonia are very common in the elderly and can reoccur a few days after the last dose of antibiotics.

Chapter Six

A stands for Ask: If a person with ADRD is able to talk then ask what's happening. Ask them questions in a gentle probing way. Inquire as to how they are feeling and what they need and you may easily discover the "why" behind the behaviour.

In many cases, in a long-term care setting, I have witnessed staff who have forgotten to ask a person with ADRD these types of questions. It appears they have relied on assumptions of their own even when the patient was clearly able to verbally communicate. There were times when the staff's assumptions were wrong. I too have found it tempting to come up with my own conclusions and not ask "why." It can be such a simple step for a caregiver to omit. For example, I had an eye opener when I finally asked someone why they were angry at another co-resident. I had assumed it was because the lady in question was sitting in the chair the angry resident normally sat in. Yet, to my dismay, when I asked the resident why she was angry she told me it was because, "She tried to steal my purse last night!" My assumption regarding the reason behind the resident's anger was erroneous because I had neglected to ask "why."

There will be situations when you may not be able to understand the individual or they may no longer be able to verbally communicate or express themselves. This is where you will need to rely on other ways to gather the Ph.A.C.T.S. Here is a list of suggestions (short, simple, to-the-point questions) to be presented in a calm caring voice:

- Are you hungry?
- Would you like a snack?
- Are you thirsty?
- Are you in pain?
- Where do you hurt?
- Do you have a headache?
- Do you hurt here? (Point or touch area on you or them)
- Do you need a nurse?
- Do you need a doctor?

- Are you worried?
- What are you worried about?
- Are you scared?
- What can I do to help you?
- What are you scared about?
- Did anyone upset you? Who?

C stands for Consider Cognitive Concerns: Consider that there is something going on in their mind that is bothering them and thus the reason behind the behaviour. You really want to consider their feelings in this moment. Put yourself into their shoes and imagine some of the normal cognitive concerns that anyone might have that could cause anxious behaviour or fears. Once again, the "Memory Onion" analogy will help your imagination.

Could they be concerned about money? This is a common one. Often those with later stages of ADRD in care homes think they don't have enough money to pay for their next meal? Perhaps they may be worried about needing to get supper ready for another family member? Could they be concerned with where to find the closest washroom? How about feelings of being pressured or threatened?

Often I have witnessed concerns for a young child, such as worries about needing to go to pick up the child from school or worries related to a perceived need to get home in time to make supper for their working husband.

Keep in mind that even though their needs are now being looked after by you, their caregiver, this does not mean their worries are erased. Often these cognitive concerns may not be what we expect the person with ADRD to worry about, because in our reality their concerns don't seem to make immediate sense. Yet, as caregivers, sensitivity is required in order to be a good detective. Failing to be observant and perceptive may result in prolonged or increased unusual or difficult behaviours.

Here are some examples of common feelings or cognitive concerns:

Chapter Six

- Worry for someone or something
- Worried about being late
- Worried about upsetting or disappointing others
- Humiliation
- Sadness recalled from a past situation
- Sadness of their losses
- Sadness of their physical changes
- Upset with themselves for not being able to do something
- Upset with a family member for not being there for them
- Fear of someone or that something will hurt them
- Fear of forgetting to do something

T stands for Triggers: What could be triggering the behaviour? Triggers for behaviours are often related to your approach, an object, an event, even a time of day that causes the person with ADRD to react in a specific manner. Is your grandmother afraid of a certain TV personality and starts to yell every time she sees him on TV? Does your mother cry heavily every time she sees her own mother's photograph? Does the time of day trigger a particular behaviour such as wandering because they "need to get home before it gets too dark?" Being aware that something may be triggering the behaviours will assist you to determine why the behaviour may be happening.

It can be helpful to keep a daily log or record describing the problem. Ask yourself, when and how often does the problem occur? Keeping a log may be worthwhile for more complicated circumstances. Here are some examples of possible triggers:

- Your impatience
- Your tone of voice
- Someone commanding them
- A certain time of the day
- Hearing certain words or phrases
- Hearing a song
- Loud noises

- Encountering unwanted touching
- Hallucinations (Visual, Touch, Taste, Sounds, Smells)
- A stranger in the room
- Crowds
- Attempting tasks they find difficult
- Certain objects
- Animals/pets
- Seeing a certain family member
- Seeing an outside door
- Seeing a car
- Seeing a certain picture
- Seeing their purse, coat, hat, wallet, shoes, etc.

S stands for Scan the environment: Look around you, and scan the physical environment; is it too noisy or maybe too quiet? Do you notice the temperature in the room is too hot or too cold for the person with ADRD? Problems relating to physical environment can turn out to be as simple as reducing the clutter or moving the ottoman. Sometimes, a crowded room can lead to upset and frustration and result in you being on the receiving end of an aggressive episode. Further, if you have scanned the environment, you can address and maybe even avoid many events that could cause behavioural issues in the first place. For example, Christmas meal at Aunt Betty's home with fifteen grandchildren all under the age of ten may no longer be the ideal party for your mom to attend, as the physical environment may be upsetting for her.

By scanning the environment, you may discover answers to "why" the person with ADRD is acting in a particular way, and what's causing it. Here are some suggestions for scanning the environment:

- Look at what the person was just doing
- Look where they were just sitting/standing
- Look to where and what their eyes are focused on

Chapter Six

- Could it be another person doing something in the room that upset them?
- Is the room too hot/cold?
- Is the room too quiet and boring?
- Is the room too stimulating and loud?
- Look for others in the room and observe their behaviour
- Ask others if they know what may have triggered the person with ADRD to become upset if you were not there

> **Helpful Hint:** Put yourself in their shoes.

Recap: To understand why the behaviour is happening, we first need to gather the **Ph.A.C.T.S.™**:
Ph - Physical?
A - Ask Them!
C - Consider Cognitive Concerns
T - Triggers?
S - Scan the Environment

Passing off the behaviour as "just their dementia/disease" or that "they are doing this on purpose" is not doing you or them any good. You are missing the opportunity to get to the root of the problem, which will help you to better come up with solutions. If you truly believe there is a reason for the behaviour (the Dementia Code) and ask yourself "why." Your brain will amaze you at how fast the wheels will turn to gather the Ph.A.C.T.S.™. If you don't ask yourself "why," then yes, managing the behaviour will not come easy to you. Asking "why" is the first step to get your critical thinking ability moving. You are now halfway there to effectively managing the behaviours. Before we move on to the next step, let's practice a little.

Enhancing Learning: Case Study

Clarence was diagnosed with middle stage Alzheimer's disease. He often wanted to go home, but the problem was, he was already home. He was living in a long-term care facility in Ontario where I was working. Day in and day out, he had his meals and slept there. However, after breakfast, most mornings, he would get very agitated and anxious. He would wheel himself in his wheelchair towards any door he could get to, pushing people out of the way in order to try and leave. Staff members would consistently explain that he was already home and did not need to leave.

It became increasingly difficult to witness Clarence become increasingly upset about his restrictions. Most staff genuinely did not know how to properly help Clarence. I knew there had to be a way to help him. I decided to put on my detective hat to find out "why?" Remember, if you do not ask yourself this very important question, your brain will not automatically go into problem solving mode.

Let's start off with a little background about wandering. It is common for people with Alzheimer's disease to wander. They will want to leave or wander away for a variety of reasons. Therefore, every situation will be unique. Some common reasons for wandering include attempting to search for someone, wanting to go home to a place they recall in their past (use the "Memory Onion" analogy), anxiety about something that is not obviously apparent (use detective hat, or "Memory Onion" analogy), disorientation about the physical environment (scan the environment), boredom, restlessness, feeling pain, or feeling uncomfortable.

Often, when working in long-term care homes, I will be informed of a situation where an individual wanted to leave. As in this case example of Clarence, I asked, "why do you think the resident wants to leave?" I often received the answer, "well, of course he wants to go home just like everyone else who lives here."

Chapter Six

At this point in the discussion, I would take that assumption a step further. I thought, okay, so the resident wants to go home, but this is where the detective work needs to go a little deeper. I invariably thought, "what does the resident want to do when they get home?" By digging deeper I was usually able to truly find out "why" and then I was able to help my co-workers to understand the "how" and we would be better able to help the resident. For Clarence, I was determined to help him but first I needed to understand why he was behaving this way. There had to be a reason so I gathered the **Ph.A.C.T.S.™**.

Physical: I didn't see any physical reason for Clarence wanting to leave. He had already eaten breakfast and had been to the washroom. He did not appear hurt, uncomfortable, or in pain.
Ask: I asked him why he wanted to go home and he easily told me. It wasn't difficult to get the answer out of him. I will reveal his answer in a few moments.
Consider Cognitive Concerns: In my initial detective work, there seemed to be a concern going on in Clarence's mind. He certainly felt he needed to get home. It made sense after I heard his answer.
Triggers: I looked for the triggers. All I could come up with was that this behaviour often happened in the mornings after breakfast.
Scan the Environment: The environment appeared to be calm and not overly stimulating. There didn't seem to be anything strange about it to me at the time. However, later I realized the environment had a lot to do with his behaviour.

Subsequent to my Ph.A.C.T.™ gathering, the answer for why he wanted to leave emerged. The answer Clarence gave me when I asked him "what do you need to do when you get home Clarence?" was "I need to get home to milk the cows!"

It all made sense now! Clarence was in a different layer of his "Memory Onion" than the staff working at the long-term care home were able to ascertain from their current reality. He believed he was back in his younger days, when he did milk cows on his family's farm, and he was showing anxious behaviour (or having a cognitive concern) about something he needed to do that was very real to him.

Upon further reflection, it is easy to understand why the trigger occurred after breakfast each morning. Most farming men will eat their breakfast and then head outside to do the faming chores. Also, in Clarence's case, ironically, he sat in a dining room that had windows that overlooked a field with horses. The environment provided an added trigger when he saw the farm animals each morning.

Now that we have our answer as to why Clarence wanted to leave the home, it is now time to take off our detective hat and get creative!

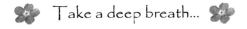

Chapter 7

Cracking Down and Getting Creative!

"There is no limit to the amount of good you can do if you don't care who gets the credit."
Ronald Reagan

Managing behaviours of those with later stages starts with identifying the possible reasons why the behaviour is happening. The process includes trying to be proactive and prevent, modify or change the behaviours into ones that are more predictable, or manageable.

First, we use our imaginary detective hat to gather the Ph.A.C.T.S.™ to help us figure out why the behaviour is happening. Then once we have determined the why (or at least a probable why), it is now time to take off the detective hat and put on our creative hat!

Creative Non-Drug Therapies

In the 2004 study mentioned previously in chapter four titled "Non-pharmacological Interventions in Dementia," by Simon Douglas, Ian James, Clive Ballard the researchers mention several non-pharmacological interventions for behaviours. They include: Behavioural therapy, Reality orientation, Validation therapy, Reminiscence therapy, Art therapy, Music therapy, Activity therapy, Complementary therapy, Aromatherapy, Bright-light therapy, Multisensory approaches, Cognitive-Behavioural therapy, and Interpersonal Therapy.

Since 1995, I have been implementing several of the non-pharmacological interventions mentioned in this study. Below is a list of the therapies that I have been using to manage behaviours for those in later stages of ADRD. To assist in encouraging you to try them as well, I have added some of my own ideas under each heading.

Validation Therapy: Naomi Feil was the developer of Validation® in the 1960s. The Validation Training Institute, Inc. advocates that rather than trying to bring the person with ADRD back to our reality, it is more positive to enter their reality. In this way empathy is developed with the person, building trust, and a sense of security. This in turn reduces anxiety. Many caregivers report increased benefits for themselves, as well as for the person with dementia, from a reduced number of conflicts and a less stressful environment.

Several of the validation principles still hold true today. Authors C. Siviero, G. Cipriani through the Congresso Nazionale di Psicologia dell'Invecchiamento, conducted research in 2011 on the Validation Method titled "Validation Method: an innovative technique for communication that permits a dignified relationship with aged disoriented people and a significant reduction of behaviour disorders." Their objective was to demonstrate the effectiveness of the validation method for the management of a case of dementia. Their report concluded, "Validation has proved to be an effective instrument for the reduction of behaviour disorders joined to dementia."

Validating someone's feelings with later stages of ADRD is a great first step in approaching someone to attempt to soften their mood. According to The Validation Training Institute, Inc. website:

> *"When one can 'step into the shoes' of another human being and 'see through their eyes,' one can step into the world of disoriented very old people and understand the meaning of their sometimes bizarre behavior."*

Interpersonal Therapy: This type of approach requires a caregiver to show empathy, sympathy, and interest while interacting with a person with ADRD. Smiles and eye contact are vital to

Chapter Seven

help build trust and acceptance, while correct use of body language and the spoken word will prevent the person with ADRD from being hurt.

Ultimately, you want to create a sense of comfort. If the opportunity presents itself, and it feels safe and appropriate, try touching a hand, or rubbing a back. Be sure your body language is giving the "I don't want to hurt you" vibe in all situations. The individual you are interacting with will be watching your body language and trying to decipher what it means.

Be convincing! You want to convince the person with ADRD that "I'm here to help you because I care." Jolene Brackey captures this topic best throughout her book titled Creating Moments of Joy published in 2007. She suggests, "Look beyond the wall of this disease and focus on the person who needs you. Love and care with a genuine heart. That is when you will fly, feel warmth, and start smelling the daisies."

> **Helpful Hint:** Ultimately, you want to create a sense of comfort.

Activity Therapy: Activity enjoyment is often dependant on the past interests of an individual along with their current abilities and skills. There are various fun activities to choose from such as listening to music, dancing, doing puzzles together, sorting (anything!), helping with the cooking, or cleaning. The list really is endless. Ideally, you want to be sure to personalize the activity to match their abilities and interest, especially in times of upset. This will be most effective in order to keep their mind off negative or upsetting concerns.

If you know of a particular trigger that will bring about certain difficult behaviour, then be proactive and engage the individual in an activity prior and during the trigger. For example, you know that the person with ADRD becomes anxious when the cleaning lady is in the house; therefore, suggest a walk or a drive for ice cream to get her out of the house until the cleaning has taken place. Another suggestion, requiring a lower scale of movement, may be to look at a puppy magazine together. Sometimes it is really all about the person with ADRD needing quality one-on-one attention for a change.

The book *Activities Keep Me Going* by Charles W. Peckham and Arline B. Peckham is a guidebook for activity personnel who plan, direct, and evaluate activities with older persons. It was one of the books that were recommended to students when I was in my first college program. In the introduction it states, "Activity gives meaning to life, adds life to years and may make the difference between the will to engage or disengage."

When providing activity ideas here are some general ideas that we often consider for those with ADRD as part of our Cognitive Massage Therapy Program™:

- **Physical exercise:** Going for a walk, attending an exercise class, going swimming, involving them in simple household chores, such as folding towels, dusting, sweeping, knitting, rolling yarn, drying dishes, and caring for plants in a garden. These common household chores help to enhance feelings of usefulness and self-worth especially for the women who were homemakers.
- **Intellectual stimulation:** Doing brain games and other mentally stimulating activities (as mentioned in chapter two).
- **Socialization:** Being with people such as getting out of the house to go for a walk in the park, going to a community centre, visiting a mall, going to parties or picnics.
- **Emotional expression:** Gardening, listening to music, and visits with children and/or pets.
- **Spiritual expression:** Practicing a religion, saying prayers, reading spiritual books, listening or singing hymns, attending spiritual community gatherings, and meditating.

While on the topic of activity therapy, it is best to incorporate a daily exercise routine. This may include a walk to the end of the street and back at the same time each day or even a few times each day depending on individual abilities. By ensuring a person with ADRD gets enough exercise and participates in a wide variety of interesting activities, many unwanted behaviours associated with boredom or restlessness may be avoided.

Activities involving music can bring about a positive and instant mood change for anyone. This can be done just by listening to a familiar music CD or even singing. Try changing a stale mood to a more positive one by saying, "I have this song stuck in my head and I can't seem to get it out. Has that ever happened to you?" Then start to hum or sing the song "you are my sunshine, my only sunshine." See how fast this one verse can lighten everyone's mood!

In some cases, you may want to have a familiar CD on hand. With a disk player handy, you can play the CD as needed to regulate the mood and maintain a positive atmosphere. If you know the afternoon brings on more behaviours and have had success with music, then perhaps you may play the same CD as a daily routine.

Recently I came across a new activity program called The Java Music Club, a program that is all about residents helping residents. Here is information about the program provided by Kristine Theurer, MA (Gerontology), MTA, the founder, Java Music Club Inc.:

> *"Java Music Club is the first standardized mutual support group activity program, specifically designed to target loneliness and depression within the long-term care sector. It is the only psychosocial program of its kind that addresses the emotional and mental health needs of residents—no musical abilities are required to facilitate the program. It is called the Java Music Club as not too many people want to attend a psychosocial mutual support intervention program, but are intrigued by the idea of a fun social group that involves coffee and music."*

The focus of this program is on residents helping residents and it provides a structure for them to seek out and support those that are lonely and isolated. It is being implemented in retirement and assisted living homes, care homes (including memory care), and adult day centres and is supported by the Ontario Association of Residents' Councils. It is structured so that staff can engage and support those with cognitive impairment using the program's tools, which include a unique combination of themes, photography, music, readings, and a traditional talking stick.

The program has been researched and the findings published in the peer-reviewed Journal of Applied Gerontology. Kristine states, "Group participants report a decrease in loneliness, an increased sense of belonging and empowerment and the development of new friendships. Once the program is established an add-on program called the Java Mentorship Program, can be implemented which helps residents seek out and support those that are lonely or isolated. Helping residents help one another."

Music Therapy: Music as a therapy is a very different approach then just listening to music. Several studies have reported that music therapy provides many benefits to persons with ADRD and behaviours. After six weeks of music therapy, one study concluded by the Department of Communication & Psychology, Aalborg University (Apr, 2013) revealed that this type of therapy reduced agitation disruptiveness and prevented medication increases in people with dementia by Simon Douglas, Ian James, Clive Ballard (2004)."

"Activities such as drawing and painting are thought to provide individuals with the opportunity for self-expression and the chance to exercise some choice in terms of the colours and themes of their creations."

Accredited Music Therapist, Brian Deo from Van-Art Expression located in British Columbia, defines music therapy as:

Chapter Seven

"Music is many things. It is a bookmark for memories both triumphant and tragic, a stimulator to encourage movement and creativity, a decelerator to calm and focus, and a backdrop for creating various moods. Although music is an easy game to 'plug and play' the levels are infinite so the game never ends. Music therapy spontaneously focuses music to suit these purposes specific to the client regardless of age, ability, or gender."

I have personally witnessed Brian helping seniors to bring back welcomed memories by playing the songs from long ago regardless of their level of cognitive impairment. Observing the unbelievable smiles is nothing short of amazing!

Art Therapy: Art therapy has been recommended as a treatment for people with dementia as it has the potential to provide meaningful stimulation, improve social interaction, and improve levels of self-esteem as stated in the study "Non-pharmacological Interventions in Dementia."

Activities such as drawing and painting are thought to provide individuals with the opportunity for self-expression and the chance to exercise some choice in terms of the colours and themes of their creations. Many people who are registered Art Therapists do in-home visits or will also visit someone in a care home. If an individual previously enjoyed creating art but is not in the position to hire an Art Therapist, then perhaps a caregiver can offer the person with ADRD tools to make art. Creating artwork may guide the individual into a different frame of mind that is creative and calm.

Reminiscence Therapy: I love reminiscing! I am sure you do as well. The same goes for someone who has a poor short-term memory but an excellent long-term memory! As discussed in the "Memory Onion" analogy, most individuals with ADRD have an enhanced ability to recall long term, rather than short-term memories. Bring up any positive topic about their past, such as where they grew up, any family pets, berry picking, making jams, hair and clothing fashion, cars they drove in, and the list goes on. Asking and actively listening to these past experiences from an individual with ADRD will make them feel great! Feel free to use images and read old short stories to get things started. Old pictures from their albums or even exploring the great stories found on the website www.reminisce.com.

Through reminiscing with a companion, an individual with ADRD has somebody who can truly go into his or her reality, even for a short moment. This activity may create a bond and build trust between the two of you. Need a way to introduce reminiscing? Why not start by saying, "you know, there is this song that I heard today, I am not sure if you have heard of it. It is called, Bicycle Built for Two. Oh you have heard of it! I really like it, would you sing it with me? I think it starts off as, Daisy, Daisy, here is my answer true..." I am certain by now they may have finished the song for you. Then, once the song concludes, you can ask to be told of a time when the person with ADRD saw a bicycle for two or if they ever were on one. In addition, you can ask if they can recall the first time they rode a bicycle. The conversation may then lead to talking about their first car or even to reminiscing about horse and carriage rides and other memorable activities. I'm sure you now get the point. Enjoy!

> **Helpful Hint:** These creative ideas for managing behaviours do work!

The following is the list of non-drug approaches that I have used and continue to incorporate into my business Personalized Dementia Solutions.

- Validation
- Interpersonal Therapy
- Therapeutic Reasoning™
- Re-Direction
- Activity Therapy

- Music
- Art
- Reminiscing Therapy
- Address Physical Needs
- Make Environmental Changes

Here follows a description of the basic principles of four other non-pharmacological approaches that I have been using since 1995, which are not included in the 2004 study by Simon Douglas, Ian James, and Clive Ballard.

Re-direction: This is a strategy that many professional caregivers have been taught over the past few decades. This method works great, but only if done properly. It is most successful when the redirection is aimed at the interests of the specific resident as is implied in the book, "Creating Successful Dementia Care Settings - Volume Three: Minimizing Disruptive Behaviors" published in 2001 by authors Kristin Perez, OTR/L; Mark A. Proffitt, M.Arch; and Margaret P. Calkins, M.Arch., Ph.D.

Ideally, you will have first exercised validation and demonstrated excellent interpersonal therapy before trying to redirect or change the topic. Try redirecting a woman two seconds after she asked you for help to find her lost young daughter by asking her to go and have a cup of coffee with you! A redirect, for this emotional circumstance, may not work without the prior use of other types of therapies and/or approaches.

Make Environmental Changes: A caregiver can remove or add things to the environment to change behaviour and remove triggers. For example, if a person with ADRD is getting upset and you notice they are in an area where it is too noisy, you may want to lead them to a quieter area.

To provide a second example, some families have a coat rack by their front door and this may prompt the person with ADRD to continually ask to leave with their coat and shoes so visible by the door. Removing these items from the environment may reduce the desire for them to want to leave.

To provide a third example, supposing there are many power tools visible in the carport or in the backyard. These tools were previously used often, but it now is no longer safe for them to operate. Perhaps it is time to use the old 'out of sight out of mind' technique to end any debate between the two of you on whether the person with ADRD can or cannot perform the power tool work.

Address Physical Needs: When discussing the gathering of the Ph.A.C.T.S.™, it was clear that much behaviour is a result of a physical issue such as pain or discomfort. It is important to be sensitive to these issues. If we detect something physical going on, we should immediately address these needs. Sometimes, if the person with ADRD is not able to communicate as well as they did previously, they will call for help in other forms. For example, if someone needs to use the toilet but is not sure where to find the toilet you may observe agitation. Perhaps this would be a great time to caringly guide the person towards the washroom area.

It would be ideal to anticipate physical needs before they arise. For example, it will be obvious after being around a person with ADRD who has spent a few hours sitting in a wheelchair that this person will benefit from some stretches or standing and sitting exercises. In addition, if a person is continually sitting in a wheelchair, it is important to ensure their seating is comfortable. I know of one situation where an individual was continually trying to get out of his wheelchair. It was discovered by an Occupational Therapist that the resident was sitting on his seat cushion backwards!

In other cases, physical needs may need to be addressed through pain medication or medication related to other conditions, such as diabetes, arthritis, thyroid, or even a vitamin deficiency. If you suspect pain, a doctor or specialist may need to be consulted

Chapter Seven

when you are not able to get to the bottom of it using your detective hat to gather the Ph.A.C.T.S.™.

Therapeutic Reasoning™: Do you recall the dictionary definition provided earlier for the word manage? You may already be aware that reasoning with someone with ADRD is not always possible. Ultimately, when using Therapeutic Reasoning™ you say, or do, anything within reason to provide the person you are caring for with reassurance. This may be the most important and the most effective creative approach you may want to use on a daily basis to assist in managing behaviours. More in-depth information and examples on this creative therapy is provided in a chapter of its own.

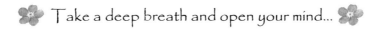 Take a deep breath and open your mind...

Chapter 8
Therapeutic Reasoning™

"No one is useless in this world who lightens the burdens of another."
Charles Dickens

Anything that is therapeutic provides a benefit. In the Online Etymology Dictionary, reasoning is defined as the mental powers concerned with forming conclusions, judgements, or inferences. Reasoning with a person who has impairment with their judgment and thinking (especially in later stages of ADRD) is not always easy.

Therapeutic Reasoning™ is a term that I have been using for many years to describe an approach to managing behaviours in later stages of ADRD. It is all about reasoning with someone with ADRD in their reality in order to have a positive outcome or benefit for all concerned. It involves using reasoning (verbal or non-verbal), which is logical to the person (not necessarily in actuality), and it creates a calm feeling. As a result, this approach can be extremely beneficial in reducing stress both for the person with ADRD and the caregiver. Although it is an effective way to manage challenging behaviours in later stages please keep in mind that this approach should only be used in limited situations. We certainly don't want to use this approach to cause harm.

Over the years I have witnessed many family and paid caregivers using this creative reasoning approach to help care for someone in later stages of ADRD. Several caregivers have told me that they would not know how they would have coped without it. Several times on my journey I have seen caregivers (especially new ones to the role) not aware of this approach. My hope is that all caregivers will be aware of all the options available to them and they will make their own choices around which approach and coping strategy to use.

It was an amazing experience for me when speaking with Ann Carlsen, an intellectual property lawyer in Burnaby BC, about my recent trademarks. When in her office explaining the concept of my book and the term Therapeutic Reasoning™, she proceeded to inform me of her past experiences of caring of her father with dementia. After hearing the approach behind Therapeutic Reasoning™ she stated to me, "It would have been such a comfort knowing there is an approach like this that would have reduced my father's stress as well as my family's stress."

> **Helpful Hint:** Would you rather be right or be at peace?

I cannot stress enough that we need to go into their reality if it appears impossible to gently encourage them into our reality. We need to say or do anything that will help them to become more at ease (not harm). We do this because we care. Therapeutic Reasoning™ is a helpful creative non-pharmacological approach to assist with reducing stress and managing behaviours that is done from a place of caring, not a place of hurtful deception.

Keeping the Peace

When reasoning becomes difficult, the goal becomes less about who is right and who is wrong. Instead the goal is to ensure everyone is happy and at peace by using the influence of tact. Irene Iris Barnes wrote a book in 2007 called Musings from a Dementia Unit. This book has many stories that help her readers foster learning from people with Alzheimer's disease. In the book she states:

> *"Caregivers need to understand the reality of those suffering from dementia, help them make sense of situations and calm their fears. It takes courage on the part of staff to step out of the medical model of caregiving into the caring model."*

Chapter Eight

This can be done by showing genuine respectful acceptance of their thoughts, feelings, and stories. It is important to be careful to respond in a way that makes sense to them. We should try our best to avoid saying things that are not true; however, in some cases you may need to put on your acting hat on top of your creative hat to effectively bring peace.

> **Helpful Hint:** Remember the definition of Manage:
> - To bring about or succeed in accomplishing, sometimes despite difficulty or hardship.
> - To dominate or influence (a person) by tact, flattery, or artifice.
>
> –www.dictionary.com

Agree: Keep the peace by using tact. What if someone firmly believes the city they are living in is Edmonton, but in reality, you are both sitting in chairs in Ontario. You may try to gently interject, "Oh, I thought we are in Ontario right now," or "Could it be that we are in Ontario?" If the individual with ADRD feels confident you are both in Edmonton, then it may be best to not argue or correct. It will be evident that the person is not willing to change their mind, so what would be the point? In fact, by refraining from correction, you will be creating, by omission, the illusion that you agree with them. Why not create this illusion? Who is it really hurting?

Apologize: Once again you are helping to keep the peace. If an individual is upset because they believe you moved something that belongs to them, your apology utilizes diplomacy to settle their agitation. When someone apologizes, this calming gesture may provide the individual with ADRD a feeling of the agitation being over with. You are going to provide a benefit to everyone concerned by using Therapeutic Reasoning™ in this way. This approach may not be easy at first, because our ego likes to kick in by telling our brain "why should I have to apologize?" Again, would you rather be right or would it be more beneficial to simply provide the apology in order to move on?

Say something nice: With this strategy you are managing behaviour by using flattery to ensure a more positive or successful outcome. Who doesn't like to hear nice things about themselves? A positive result is likely to occur when you enter a room, smile, and tell the person with ADRD, that they look nice today. Instead of saying, "Oh my! Mom, why are you wearing your shirt on backwards?" It may be wise to start out with a compliment, rather than a non-flattering approach especially if you were hoping to convince mom to get into the shower—something she has been refusing to do lately. Your goal is to create a positive vibration, which encourages feelings of acceptance and trust so you can effectively manage the behaviour.

Actively listen then verbalize you will look into it: This type of creative Therapeutic Reasoning™ has had lots of success. Often an individual with ADRD may just need to vent. I know there are times when I need to vent to a girlfriend, which doesn't necessarily mean I expect a solution to my problem in that moment. Why would it be any different for someone with ADRD? Why not give it a test try?

If you are approached with an angry issue, or a complaint about a situation or another person, then actively listen. After doing so, you may need to ask, "Do you want me to look into this for you?" If the answer is yes, demonstrate with conviction that you will need some time but you will look into the matter. Watch how their body language changes. If they are presenting a calmer demeanour, then you did your job. There was benefit for all!

In the event you are approached about your duty to look into that particular matter, you have two choices. You may switch on the Therapeutic Reasoning™ approach again by apologizing for forgetting and reassure you will try again tomorrow. Or you may want to actually look into the situation for them as promised, as it may be relevant and necessary.

Chapter Eight

> **Helpful Hint:** We as caregivers need to go into the world of the person with ADRD if they are no longer able to understand actual reality.

Learn the art of letting go: Other than times that are not safe, you may need to learn the phase, "So what?" So what if they are wearing their pyjamas inside out? So what they are making a mess trying to eat their potato salad? So what they are taking and hiding all the spoons? So what they are messing up their closet?

One other common example to share would be, "So what if they are not able to take a full bath today?" Perhaps they are now in a stage where it is going to be easier to wash their body in stages on different days. This is often related to in long-term care as a one-week bath. These are simply a few examples to provide some ideas of the types of issues that may be applicable for a caregiver to let slide. It may be hard to let go at first but with some practice you may find yourself feeling less stress as a result.

Putting Therapeutic Reasoning™ to Practice

Once again the goal, or purpose, of using Therapeutic Reasoning™ is to keep the peace, and manage difficult behaviours to create a beneficial result for everyone involved.

Some people with ADRD may experience delusions or hallucinations. Delusions are false perceptions that are held with absolute conviction, are not changed by a compelling argument or proof to the contrary, and are patently untrue. An example of a delusion would be when a person with ADRD accuses a person of stealing from them or trying to poison them, when everybody else knows this is totally implausible. Hallucinations involve false messages being received from any of the five senses: seeing, hearing, tasting, feeling, and smelling. The person who is hallucinating sees, hears, tastes, feels, or smells, something that is not really there. An example of a hallucination would be when a person with ADRD demonstrates they are seeing a child in the room, who nobody else can see, or indicate that they are hearing noises in the room that nobody else can hear. It is important to understand these experiences can be quite vivid and upsetting to a person with ADRD.

To assist you in these circumstances and this suggestion comes from my own experience, start with asking simple questions to determine whether the experience is causing any upset or anxiety. Then, after you obtain enough information you can then tailor your responses to guide the person with ADRD into a mood of feeling at ease. Some caregivers may try to re-orient the person with ADRD back to reality by informing them that the delusions or hallucinations are not valid or real. I have seen more success in redirecting their attention and in some ways down-playing the situation if these delusions or hallucinations are not causing undue upset or anxiety to the person with ADRD who is experiencing them. For example I may ask, "Are the people in this room causing you upset?" If they respond by saying, "No," then I may say, "Well, that is good news. However, make sure you tell me if they do start to bother you and we will look into making sure they stop." Just by showing you care and want to assist can help them to feel more in control.

Another common behavioural issue occurs when a person with ADRD becomes agitated when they have a delusion that a parent or family member is worried about their whereabouts. It is helpful to remember the "Memory Onion" analogy when working through this type of behavioural occurrence. For example, Tom who lived in an Alzheimer Unit approached me out of the blue asking if his mom knew he would not be coming home for supper tonight. I initially provided some interpersonal therapy and validated his concerns by saying, "Well it sounds like you don't want your mom to worry." Since I knew Tom and I knew he would of have not been able to come to our reality, I decided to try a little Therapeutic Reasoning™. I informed him that we would contact his mother to let her know we were

Chapter Eight

providing him with supper tonight. He seemed very pleased and relieved. Once he heard this, he was then guided with ease to his seat in the dining room.

There are other instances where Therapeutic Reasoning™ may be stepped up a little to provide added reassurance. This may include incorporating a little role-playing with your creative and acting hats. For example, Doris who lived in a long-term care home where I worked approached me one day looking panicked. She was wondering if she would be able to stay overnight. I told her in a reassuring voice, "Of course!" She looked at me as though she was not convinced. She repeated her request, asking me if I was certain she would be able to stay overnight. I then decided to step things up a little to reassure her to the best of my abilities. "I am almost certain Doris, but if you would like, I could look into it for you." She was now looking very pleased. I decided it was time to put on my actress hat and so I took a little walk around the corner and out of her sight, waited a few moments, and then came marching back towards her with a big grin while nodding my head saying, "Yes, they said that will not be a problem and they are happy you will be staying with us tonight." Doris let out a deep sigh and said, "Oh thank you so much!"

The following example relates to a caregiver, a husband named Dave, who was taking care of his wife, Rose in their home and needed some supports from the community. However, his wife was not amenable to strangers coming into the home to help out. Thus, Dave was at an impasse when he came to me for advice. Dave really wanted a home support worker to come into his home to help clean and to take his wife out for walks. He was really feeling the need to have some time to himself. However, his wife, Rose refused to consider the idea. She felt they did not need someone to come in to help them. Rose insisted that there was nothing wrong with her even though she was not able to keep up with the housework and was no longer able to fix meals due to her early to middle stage Alzheimer's disease.

What was Dave to do? He was feeling the added stress as a

caregiver and knew this type of support would greatly assist him in his role. After receiving some education from Personalized Dementia Solutions, it was decided he would use Therapeutic Reasoning™. He informed his wife that he had heard from a schoolteacher friend about a new girl in town from the Philippines. This girl, who was attending school, needed to find a short-term practicum placement. This requirement was part of a job-training program while she is here for a visit to Canada. (Wink, wink!) Dave explained to his wife, Rose, that this girl really needs help for only a few weeks and asks if we can "help her." Rose has a soft spot for helping others and agrees. As Maria builds a friendship with Rose and involves Rose in some of the homemaking tasks, a bond is formed. Rose forgets all about Maria's limited time in Canada and Dave continues to receive the much-needed support. The solution ends up a win-win situation for all!

Coming up with creative solutions that may not be logical to you can be awkward at first. You may not feel comfortable with these types of strategies all at once. However, once you get used to this new way of interacting with the person you are caring for, the easier it may become and the quicker you will be able to defuse unwanted behaviours.

Practice will make perfect. I have had several families approach me saying they really wished they could have been more comfortable with Therapeutic Reasoning™ from the beginning as it has now made a huge impact on their lives. Again, you are using this technique coming from a place of caring for an individual in the later stages of ADRD to assist in managing the behaviours.

> **Helpful Hint:** Don't knock Therapeutic Reasoning™ until you have tried it. Some families wish they could have been using it long before they finally surrendered to this helpful creative therapy.

Chapter Eight

Case Study Solutions

Returning to our story about Clarence, let's apply some of the above creative techniques. As we know, Clarence was reliving his younger days on the farm. After breakfast, when looking out the window of the dining room, Clarence would became anxious and attempt to leave the premises to go home to milk the cows. Knowing why he wanted to leave now helped to put things into perspective. I had to think of the best way to manage this behaviour. My strategy was to join him in his reality; I did not try to convince him of mine.

Initially, a Validation approach was provided while applying Interpersonal Therapy. Once I discovered why he wanted to leave, I said to him, "Oh, of course, I would be worried about the cows too!" All of a sudden he appeared more at ease. His body language told me that he was relieved that I understood his predicament and cared about him and his situation. However, he remained concerned. I then improvised by saying, "You know Clarence, I think the cows have already been milked today? Let me go be sure." At this point I was using Therapeutic Reasoning™ and putting on my actress hat to make it more reassuring for him.

I left the area and went behind a doorway. I waited a few moments then came back with a large smile saying, "Well, lucky us! Those cows have already been milked today! Isn't this great news!" I could tell he was pleased but needed more reassurance, because he asked me, "Are you sure?" Still wearing my actress hat, as I knew this was the best way to alleviate his concerns, I provided non-verbal affirmation by nodding my head. While smiling I provided verbal affirmation by saying, "Yes, I am sure! It was actually your brother who milked the cows. You have an amazing brother Clarence!" At this point, Clarence finally seemed totally convinced and at ease. This was the reassurance that Clarence had needed, and no longer was he actively seeking to leave the long-term care home. I was then able to use the creative approach of redirection by suggesting, "How about joining me for a cup of coffee or tea to celebrate? The treat is on me!"

 Why not take in a quick breath...

Potential Alternative to Clarence's case:

The concept of Therapeutic Reasoning™ may seem simple, and it is! However, if you don't take the time to ask yourself why or to gather the Ph.A.C.T.S.™ about a problem, it may not be easy to solve. If you think about Clarence's situation from the point of view of reality, you know he is already home. So why would you even wonder why he wants to go home? The answer is, if you don't ask, and you simply address his behaviour of trying to escape by trying to talk sense into him, or preventing him from making it to the front door, you will become exhausted and fed up.

A caregiver with minimal dementia care understanding may have responded to Clarence by taking him to his room and verbalizing to him, "Here is your room Clarence. Here are all your things. See, this is your home!" Further, if this caregiver heard Clarence say something about milking the cows, an attempt may have been made to bring him back to reality by saying, "But you don't have to milk the cows anymore Clarence because you don't live on the farm anymore. The farm is sold and you live here now."

Do you think Clarence would have accepted these comments, from the above caregiver if he was firmly in a past layer of his "Memory Onion?" While it is very possible to bring an individual in the early stages of ADRD back to our reality, it becomes less possible as the disease progresses. Unfortunately, many individuals in later stages of ADRD will never be able to come back to our reality.

If after hearing comments from a caregiver in a reality that was not his, Clarence could have become very disruptive and

Chapter Eight

maybe decided that fighting a person past the door is the only way he can "get out." Often this is the time when it may be quite common to hear a staff member call out to the nurse, "I think it is time for someone's happy pill!" If this had been the result, how sad would it have been to drug Clarence? It was almost effortless to manage Clarence's behaviour by calming him down by using some creative approaches. This is because the "why" was discovered in his circumstance.

> **Helpful Hint:** We need to practice going into the reality of a person with ADRD

When difficult situations like this happen for family caregivers who are caring for a loved one with later stages of ADRD outside a long-term care home, rest assured the same creative therapy approaches can also apply. Just be sure to remember that since all behaviour has meaning, you will need to first seek the Ph.A.C.T.S.™ before you put on your creative hat to come up with a solution that meets their needs.

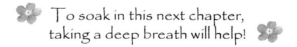
To soak in this next chapter,
taking a deep breath will help!

Chapter 9

Approach, Approach, Approach!

"He that can have patience can have what he will."
Benjamin Franklin

Approach. Your approach is ultimately the best way to manage behaviours! Your approach means everything! It is very common for someone with ADRD to mirror you and your attitude. Therefore you want to be sure you are sending the right messages both verbally and non-verbally.

As indicated earlier in the book, it really all boils down to the Golden Rule: "do unto others as you would have them do unto you." Be kind, gentle, understanding, supportive, helpful, fun to be around, respectful, caring, and sensitive. You need to be the peacekeeper now and want to avoid confrontation as much as you can in each moment.

Gentle Caring Approaches

Providing gentle caring approaches when you are looking to provide care or seek the assistance of a person with ADRD will go a long way towards gaining their trust and allowing them to feel comfortable with you. I am proud to say I have been certified in GPA (Gentle Persuasive Approaches) since 2006 and as of 22 May 2013, I am now certified as a Canadian GPA trainer for AGE: Advanced Gerontological Education. To learn more about GPA training, please see the GPA website at, www.ageinc.ca.

> **Helpful Hint:** Be a peacekeeper!

"Greet before you treat" is a well-known line by Teepa Snow, MS, OTR/L, FAOTA a Dementia Care Specialist located in the

USA who trains and consults for agencies, facilities, and families. Teepa also created a video in collaboration with a company in the USA called Senior Helpers. In this video Teepa describes the different stages of dementia called the "Senior Gems". She uses different gems to describe the abilities and how as caregivers we need to provide the right type of care and environment for that particular gem. I highly suggest watching this video as learning other angles of how to provide good care can only help us to be better caregivers.

In my opinion, the line by Teepa Snow "greet before you treat" should be memorized and rehearsed by all who are caregivers. If we do not greet before we treat, we can easily be the ones who triggered the behaviour in the first place. In fact, many times our attitude, our approach our tone and our poor communication techniques can contribute to the behaviours in the first place.

> **Helpful Hint:** Greet before you treat!

Person-Centred Approach

The focus of person-centred approach is on the person rather than on the illness or the disabilities. Psychologist Dr. Carl Rogers (1902-1987) developed the Person-Centred Approach. Rogers' theory and work is very simple to describe yet "it can be very difficult to put into practice because the approach does not use techniques but rather relies on the personal qualities of the therapist/person (caregivers) to build a non-judgemental and empathic relationship," according to the website of the British Association for the Person-Centred Approach.

To provide a person-centred approach, it is important to know the person you are caring for. This includes their likes, dislikes, and personality. This is where I like to refer to the quote by Hippocrates, "It's far more important to know what person the disease has than what disease the person has." Not only will it help you to discover quicker if something is physically going on with the person you are caring for, you will also be able to develop a closer bond. It can also be extremely helpful in becoming aware of their warning signs of behaviours that indicate frustration, anxiety, and even aggression related to triggers. Of course when you notice these behaviours starting to surface, it is in both your best interest (and the others who will be interacting with them the rest of the day) to do what you can to prevent or reduce the possible causes.

In the book Gentle Care by Moyra Jones she discusses a technique called Behaviour Mapping. This technique is useful for caregivers to better understand the daily pattern of a person with ADRD. It involves doing an observation over a 24-hour period to determine the percentage of time a person is sleeping, walking, at rest, doing an activity, etc. This technique could be useful to you in your role as a detective.

> **Helpful Hint:** In person-centred care, learn what makes them happy, then provide it!

In chapter four, we discussed a coping possibility of taking a break and trying again later. This helpful approach will allow some breathing time between tasks and may make a huge difference in lowering the frustrations of a person with ADRD. The last thing you want is for someone to become so upset that they become aggressive towards you or others. Doing what we can to keep them calm is best. Taking a breather by stepping back from the situation to reassess what you need to do next is a great plan.

For paid caregivers who work in long-term care, it is in your best interest to read over the "Guidelines for Care: Person-centred care of people with dementia living in care homes framework" that was produced by the Alzheimer Society of Canada in 2011. This guideline covers a broad range of care approaches. This publication mentions the important role that families and friends have in helping the individual with ADRD have a "good day" in the care home. This can be accomplished by families sharing critical information about their loved ones likes and dislikes with the front line care staff. Doing so can assist the care staff with their daily caregiving tasks and result in a better experience for the loved one in care. The Alzheimer Society's "Guidelines for Care: Person-centred care of people with dementia living in care homes framework" states that, "people with dementia have the right to enjoy the highest possible quality of life and quality of care by being engaged in meaningful relationships which are based on equality, understanding, sharing, participation, collaboration, dignity, trust and respect." I couldn't agree more.

The Importance of Knowing the Person You are Caring For

Knowing the person you are caring for with ADRD will help you to better relate to them and support them. You will also have an easier time using creative therapies such as Therapeutic Reasoning™. It will be much easier to know how and when it may be acceptable to use role-playing to reinforce their reality. If you know the person well, and you get caught in an explanation that doesn't make sense to them, it will be less of a worry. It will be easier for you to come up with something different and apologize to regain their trust. As discussed earlier, when this happens, it is possible that they will forget your conversation shortly after anyway.

> **Helpful Hint:** Do or say whatever works!

To help you understand the importance of knowing the person you are caring for, I will share with you my story about Eve. In order to prevent Eve from leaving her long-term care unit to take a "cab home" I needed to dig deeper to understand why she wanted to leave in the first place. I gathered the Ph.A.C.T.S.™ and discovered she had a cognitive concern. She told me she wanted to go home because her welfare cheque was there and needed to be cashed. (This certainly was no longer the case.) I decided to try to use Therapeutic Reasoning™.

Chapter Nine

I asked Eve if she wanted me to ask her daughter to pick up the cheque for her, explaining that this plan would save on the cost of a cab fare. Eve looked at me with concerned eyes and asked me which daughter? Oh no, based upon the way she was staring at me, I realized I had to be sure to pick the right daughter! I decided to tell her that it was her oldest daughter who would pick up the cheque for her. This comment led her to exclaim, "No way! She is a thief and will spend it all!" Okay, so now I had to think fast! I decided to try again. "Did I say oldest? I am so sorry, I meant to say the youngest." Eve looked at me and said, "Are you sure?" Feeling a little more at ease, I replied convincingly, "Yes, I am sure." Eve appeared more calm and pleased with this suggestion. Saving money on a taxi fare is always a good idea and my offer of a free meal (as supper time was near) also made her day.

The important thing to realize here is you too may someday pick the wrong answer. Using a person-centred approach and Therapeutic Reasoning™ such as sincerely apologizing for your mistake and saying you feel it best to look into it, may prove to be most helpful.

Here is an important note for those working in care homes or for a home care company: once you, as a caregiver, have developed more understanding of the person you are caring for with ADRD and have developed strategies for managing their behaviours, it is important to share these strategies with others who are also taking care of this individual, including the family. For example, if you have discovered a solution to limiting their frustrations when you are getting them dressed, then passing this on as it will facilitate a consistent routine for the individual and of course be less frustrating for all those involved in the caregiving task.

> **Helpful Hint:** Share your solutions!

Consistent Routines

On the topic of routine, it can't be stressed enough how important it is to maintain a consistent one. Veering off even slightly from the normal routine of a person with ADRD may escalate behaviours. Can we really blame them for this? For example, how would you feel if you always had coffee before you had a shower and today someone decided to prevent you from your normal routine? This also applies when arranging for the care of someone with ADRD. It is important to keep the caregivers as consistent as possible.

Esther Heerema, MSW wrote an article called "9 Benefits of Consistent Caregivers for People with Dementia" on 25 February 2013 in the About.com Guide. In this article it mentions that a familiar paid caregiver may be more likely to prevent or diffuse behaviours successfully. She states, "More and more, facilities are leaning toward consistent caregivers for residents, especially those residents with memory loss and confusion". This is not always easy to arrange but if possible it would be ideal.

❀ You may want to take a deep breath now to help you clear your mind to absorb the message from this important next chapter. ❀

Chapter 10

Importance of Good Communication

"Good communication does not mean that you have to speak in perfectly formed sentences and paragraphs. It isn't about slickness. Simple and clear go a long way."
John Kotter

Communication allows us to express our thoughts, our wishes, and our beliefs. It also can play a major role in shaping our relationships with others. Besides providing proper approaches, practicing creative therapies, and ensuring routines, it is also imperative we utilize proper communication techniques. We can do this verbally through our words or tones, or physically through our body language and facial expressions.

By remaining sensitive and understanding about any communication difficulties that are apparent in the person we are caring for with ADRD we can effectively support them. Just as we would assist someone struggling with a physical limitation, such as someone walking on crutches through a door, we should also be supportive to someone with cognitive limitations. Keep in mind that just because we can't see the internal damage, it doesn't mean it isn't happening. ADRD causes damage to the neurons.

As mentioned in chapter four, repeated questions are very common behaviour for those with cognitive impairment. It can be very hard for caregivers to hear these questions over and over. Know that you are not alone. In these instances, a person with ADRD will truly believe they have not asked you five to ten times already. This is where we need to change our ways as caregivers. I know this is not always easy, but try taking a deep breath, and then answer their repeated question as calmly as you can. Remember, the individual with ADRD believes it is the first time they are hearing your answer. Thus, if caregivers fail to respond as if it is the first time, the individual with ADRD may become upset by an irritated tone of voice, or by body language that is unreceptive. Conflict can easily happen if we are not careful. When the challenge of repetitive questioning arises, this is a great time to remind ourselves that it is the disease at work.

One possible reason for repeated questions from my experience has been because the individual was not feeling reassured enough. In some cases it helped to have the answer to their question in written form. In other cases the individual with ADRD needed a stronger yet gentle caring response with conviction (through body language and tone of voice) for added reassurance.

Non-Verbal Communication

Actions really do speak louder than words, but the person who receives your actions has to be able to understand them. For someone who has difficulty interpreting messages inside their brain, understanding actions can be more difficult. This is where a person with ADRD could use some additional help. According to the article "Credibility, Respect, and Power: Sending the Right Nonverbal Signals" by Debra Stein:

> *"Research shows that more than 93 percent of communications effectiveness is determined by eye contact, body language, facial expression and voice quality. When you're trying to convey important messages like, 'I am telling the truth,' or, 'I respect you,' or when you're establishing the power positions of the parties, the nonverbal signals you send can be even more important than the particular words you are speaking."*

If you are trying to explain something to an individual with later stages of ADRD, why not use some gestures to help get your point across. For instance, rub your stomach when asking, "Are you hungry?" Also, be mindful about your tone as they could pick up on your tone before understanding the actual words or even your gestures.

Chapter Ten

Caregivers can also learn a lot from the body language of a person with ADRD. Once you know the hidden meaning behind their specific gestures, facial expressions, body stances, and body movements, you will be better at understanding the person you are caring for and may be better able to defuse any unwanted behaviours.

Tips for Effective Communication

Another suggestion for communicating with someone with later stages of ADRD is to never communicate the word or shake your head to suggest, "NO". It would be best to convey, "Yes, that is a good idea. How about we do ___ first then we will look at doing ___ after." Be sure to be using nonverbal expression of a smile and nodding your head up and down to show you agree. This will translate into respect and trust towards you. Even if the words are not understood, your calm body language and tone may be reassuring enough. I highly suggest coming back to this section to refresh and also to evaluate how you have been doing with your communication techniques. It is easy to slip up and forget. Practice makes perfect! These following communication points are adapted from the Alzheimer's Disease & Dementia Guide put out in Fall 2012 by a Canadian home care company called We Care Home Health Services.

Some Tips for Communicating with Someone in Early Stages of ADRD:

- Be patient
- Limit distractions as much as possible.
- Give the person time to express themselves.
- Don't interrupt.
- Be supportive.
- Don't talk about the person as if they are not there.
- Don't be condescending.

- Don't be patronizing.
- Avoid asking questions which rely on their memory
- Try communicating simple reminders by using short notes.
- Find a quiet place to talk.
- Avoid criticizing, correcting, or arguing.
- Look beyond the words they use. Watch body language to understand what the person is experiencing and/or expressing.

Some Tips When Communication Becomes More Difficult in Later Stages of ADRD:

- Approach the person calmly from the front.
- Make eye contact.
- Identify yourself clearly.
- Avoid sudden movements that may frighten them.
- Call the person by their name.
- Use short simple sentences.
- Give visual cues by pointing to the object you are talking about.
- Ask one question at a time and wait for a response.
- Ask questions which require a simple yes or no answer (Instead of saying "What would you like to wear?" ask "Would you like to wear this?")
- Limit choices you offer them such as, "Would you like to wear this or this?"
- Avoid vague words such as "Put it over there." Instead say, "Put it on the table."
- If repeating yourself, use exactly the same words again. Best not to rephrase as this can increase confusion. If the person is still not able to understand, try again with a simpler phrase.
- Ask the person to point or gesture if they can't find the right word or expression.
- Pay attention to your body language and facial expressions. Try a gentle, positive approach.

Ultimately, we want to encourage and reassure those with ADRD that they are doing well and that they are loved. We can do this verbally through our words or tones, or physically through our body language and facial expressions. I would like to reiterate that if your words are not understood especially for someone in later stages of ADRD, your calm tones might be reassuring enough.

> **Helpful Hint:** : It is best to refrain from saying the word "NO". Instead use positive words and positive body language.

Ways to Address Conflict

I wrote earlier about Brenda Hooper, a Mediator and Conflict Resolution Specialist from Step by Step Mediation Services. The second handout that Brenda provides when she speaks to family caregivers is on "Reaction to Thwarting Ploys." What the heck are Thwarting Ploys you ask? Thwarting Ploys are strategies that are meant to undermine, sabotage, and otherwise sideline us, by the person we are in conflict with. Holly Weeks is the author of, "Failure To Communicate: How conversations go wrong and what you can do to right them" and who also teaches and consults on communications issues in general.

There is a range of responses to Thwarting Ploys that one may use in conflict from one extreme of being passive or to the other extreme of being aggressive. On the passive side we can play along. Interestingly enough, "playing along" fits nicely into the coping strategy of managing the behaviour through Therapeutic Reasoning™, do nothing, or focus on the content. On the aggressive side we can impose behaviour, threaten or accuse or even punish. Where in this range are you when it comes to conflict? How about the person you are caring for?

Being aware of the more effective ways to address conflict can be very helpful during difficult situations as it relates to your role as a caregiver.

Here are some helpful phrases that I have used to help during a tense or concerning situation:

- "How can I help you?"
- "I don't blame you for feeling this way. I wouldn't like it if this happened to me. How about I look into this for you?"
- "You don't seem happy. What is it I can do to make thing better. Know that I will do my best to look into this for you."
- "Oh my, I hear what you are saying. How does this make you feel?"
- "Boy, it sure sounds like you have been busy with this situation."
- "I fully understand your reason for not being happy right now."
- "I would like to help you. How about I write it all down so I don't miss anything." (This could really help them to feel heard.)
- "I know this must be painful. How about I go really slowly and you tell me if it hurts and I will stop. I wouldn't want to see this wound get worse if we just leave it."
- "I would love to go outside today too. Let's first go take a peak out the window to see what the weather is doing before me make a decision."

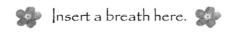
Insert a breath here.

# Chapter 11

Meaning Behind the Behaviour: Putting It Into Practice

"I don't think of all the misery, but of the beauty that still remains."
Anne Frank, The Diary of a Young Girl

Reading the stories of individuals with Alzheimer's disease and other types of dementia allows us to better understand and learn how to make their situation better. Here are some true stories that required Therapeutic Reasoning™ and several other creative techniques.

Paulette: Miscommunication (or lack of communication) will usually create confusion and lead to distress and apprehension, and making assumptions is no better. Our story follows this pattern exactly.

Imagine this: someone you can't recognize comes up to you and starts pulling off your shoes. **(Trigger)** How would you feel? You may definitely be confused, upset, and maybe angry **(Cognitive Concerns)**. Paulette's reaction was the same. Of course, Paulette is a woman with middle stage Alzheimer's disease, and the person taking off her shoes is a staff caregiver helping a podiatrist whose purpose is to examine her feet. Now that the situation is explained, you understand it, but did Paulette?

Alzheimer's disease breaks down the abstract-thinking brain function, and the natural ability to understand a situation, or to recognize the people we interact with in our daily lives. It's true that the nursing home staff and podiatrist are the types of people that Paulette interacts with on a daily basis, but her disease disables her from recognizing and even feeling totally familiar and comfortable with them.

The caregiver and the doctor assumed that Paulette understood why they were taking off her shoes; when she resisted, the care staff person said, "But you haven't had your feet done in three months!" Logically, the staff caregiver assumes Paulette will understand what is going on; podiatrist treatment she has had performed many times. It is a routine event, and Paulette should understand they would not hurt her. It should be obvious to Paulette that by taking off her shoes, they want to examine her feet. However, this is not the case. Paulette's mind cannot understand the idea of caregivers, doctors, and foot examinations. All she understands is that someone is attempting to take her shoes from her.

To investigate why Paulette was becoming fearful and upset, I got down to her eye level, where she sat, and asked how she was feeling; to my surprise she yelled, "That woman is trying to steal my shoes!" Paulette was a woman who was never financially comfortable, and her fears were founded upon her past experiences and lifestyle. To help make her feel comfortable and secure about not losing her shoes, I first validated her feelings. I then explained the reason the staff caregiver and podiatrist needed to take her shoes off to examine her feet, and I let her know that she could hold on to her shoes for the duration of the examination.

The caregiver and podiatrist's lack of communication (not explaining why they needed to take off her shoes) led to Paulette's misunderstanding of the situation. Once the situation was made clear to her, she felt comfortable enough to allow the doctor to examine her feet. With a little thoughtfulness, clear communication, and explanation of the proceedings, the podiatrist was able to carry out his work. Paulette even allowed the podiatrist to clip her toenails without a fight or struggle.

Roy: What are we afraid of when we're young? In Roy's case, his fear of being left alone was creating a disruptive problem. But Roy was not a young boy; he was a kinder and gentler older man

Chapter Eleven

in a long-term care home. His dementia related to Alzheimer's disease was gradually worsening his memory; making him fear being alone. In addition, his eyesight was very bad. This complication was not helping his situation.

Roy's fear of being alone was creating havoc at the long-term care home. In addition to calling for his mother, he would gradually become upset, which would escalate to yelling and screaming, disrupting everyone's day. **(Cognitive Concern)** He wanted someone, anyone to be with him at all times. Having someone with him would calm him. Unfortunately, companionship was not always possible; the staff had busy schedules and many other people to care for.

Roy's loneliness and fear of being alone were clear to us, but what should we do? An interesting notion occurred to me. Roy loved animals so much and since I usually brought my gentle and obedient dog to work at the long-term care home, I figured out a plan.

One day, I went over to Roy and asked him if he would like to look after my dog for me **(Activity Therapy/Distraction)** while I attended to my other duties in the nearby office. He was thrilled! He sat quietly holding tightly to the leash, feeling very useful and important, and instead of yelling out, he spoke with my dog, saying, "Nice doggy; you're such a good doggy." Even without a peep out of the dog, it was obvious that Roy felt calmed, as if someone was there beside him, listening. He felt he had good company, and he mostly loved that he had a presence of a dog because he always had a dog in his life while growing up.

This was not a long-term solution, though. I did not always bring my dog to work with me, and often on the days I didn't, Roy's fears came back and he became disruptive once again.

It was time to think creatively. With Roy's poor eyesight, we decided to try an idea to provide him comfort. **(Activity Therapy/Distraction & Therapeutic Reasoning™)** We found a large stuffed dog and put a leash on it. We brought the dog over to Roy, sat it by his leg, and gave the leash to him. I said, "Hi Roy, would you kindly look after this wonderful dog for me? I know you always do a great job at looking after dogs." As always, Roy was thrilled to help out and have the presence of something there beside him. He was not aware the dog was not real. With this new creative idea, his needs could now be met any day of the week. This creative idea worked for Roy because of his advanced dementia, poor eyesight and his love for dogs.

It's important to understand that many individuals affected by ADRD, can revert back to their childhood memories or fears like mentioned in the "Memory Onion" analogy. Thus, troublesome behavior may surface. For Roy, it was the fear of being left alone and needing familiarity. For others, it could be the fear of darkness, fear of thunderstorms, fear of losing things or even the fear of critters in the closet. As caregivers, we must be very aware and sensitive to this, and work towards coming up with creative solutions to ease their concerns in order to best manage their behaviour.

Mr. Karol: What is ability? It's having competence to do an activity. What is usefulness? It's being of service and serving a purpose. What is accomplishment? It's doing something admirably and feeling the fulfilment of that action.

Guess what's missing from a person's emotional needs when they're in the later stages of a dementia related condition/disease, including the later stages of Alzheimer disease? You guessed right, they don't feel able, useful, or a sense of fulfilment anymore. What can they do about it?

Mr. Karol regularly moved furniture in his long-term care home. **(Consider Cognitive Concern)** Unfortunately, his action (strange, and not understood by most people) was met by a negative reaction from the nurses who tried to stop him every time. Since Mr. Karol had lost his speech to Alzheimer's, he had no way of explaining his action, and since his action was instinctive rather than logical, he may not have been able to explain it if he was able to speak properly.

Chapter Eleven

As Mr. Karol was trying to lift a chair in the dining room one day, a nurse and I approached him at the same time to keep the situation safe. However, we had two different ideas of how to do this. The nurse grabbed the end of the chair and struggled to take it from him. I witnessed a molehill of a situation rapidly becoming a mountain. I quickly asked the nurse to let me handle it. She advised me to be careful, and explained that he would become violent as he always had with her. Apparently, one time he had hit her in the chest when they struggled over a similar situation. Perhaps she triggered this reaction?

I knew I had to understand why Mr. Karol was lifting chairs onto tables, but I first needed to get through this risky situation, so I stood by as he completed his action. I took the other end of the chair from the nurse, and with a very composed and calm demeanour, I gave Mr. Karol a smile **(Interpersonal Therapy)** and let him guide it toward where he wanted it to go (on top of the table). When that was over, I thanked him for his hard work, and he started to casually wander out of the dining room and down the hall as if he was happy to have done something that he deemed important. When he had gone, I took the chair back down from the table, making sure he didn't see me do this because I didn't want him to see me undoing his work and become upset.

Mr. Karol had no other incidents that day, nor was there any more aggressive assaults. I sensed that these behaviours might have stopped because he had done what he had set out to do without someone trying to stop him. After talking with his wife a few days later, I learned that Mr. Karol had worked in a grocery store, which involved lots of moving of items within the store. Likely, in his mind, he was doing a task that made him feel able, gave him a sense of accomplishment, and even perhaps made him feel useful. As explained in the "Memory Onion" analogy, I wonder if he felt it was something that had to be done because he was back in time in his past reality. **(Cognitive Concern)**

The feeling of accomplishment that comes with doing and completing a task, is natural for anyone, even for people with a dementia related condition or disease, including Alzheimer's disease. When people with dementia are allowed to do tasks according to their abilities, they feel able, useful, a sense of accomplishment, and generally good about themselves.

Take the opportunity to help those in your care to feel good by providing them with a few choices; even choices that are limited will help them feel their input is valued. Also, offer them activities they enjoy such as folding towels or gathering the napkins or dirty dishes after meals to reinforce their feelings of being able to participate and feel accomplishment.

Mary: When it comes to dealing with people who have a dementia related condition or disease, including Alzheimer's disease, a little innocent role-play may result in obtaining valuable information. This story starts with Mary, a woman with mid-to-advanced Alzheimer's disease, who had severe short memory loss, bad eyesight, and no teeth, yelling, "Doctor!" for two days' straight. **(Physical)**

Just to make sure the point is driven home, I reiterate. For two days Mary yelled for a doctor. If anyone you loved were to yell for anything, even for a few hours, you would be concerned—if you care for someone with Alzheimer's, please make sure you address them, and try to find out what it is they need; one way to do this is by asking questions.

When I found out about Mary's yelling, I went to her and asked her why she was calling for a doctor. Her answer was that she didn't want a doctor; she wanted to see a dentist. The automatic and logical answer came from a caregiver in the long-term care home, "But Mary, you don't have any teeth." I continued to question Mary, asking whether she had a problem with her teeth, and she said, "Yes." I then knew that the source of her pain must have been coming from her mouth or gums; I asked her to open her mouth so I could see and pass on the information to a dentist, but she said, "No."

It's about trust. Instinctively we know that we can trust a dentist

Chapter Eleven

to assess and treat any tooth-related ailment; this knowledge is basic and innate, because we're familiarized with it all our lives, from childhood to adulthood. It's this knowledge that Mary was using to judge her needs, and since I wasn't a dentist, she couldn't trust me to help her. It is logic boiled down to basics, and that's exactly what people like Mary, with Alzheimer's disease, use to understand the world around them—they are not capable of complex thought anymore. **(Therapeutic Reasoning™)**

Here's where it gets a little fun. That's right, you can have fun with your work. It keeps you interested and on your toes, and the person you're caring for happy. I told Mary that I would get a dentist to come to help her. A few minutes later, knowing that she would have already forgotten who I was, and with her poor eyesight would not recognize me easily, I appeared wearing a white sweater and said, "Hi Mary, I'm a dentist; how can I help you?"

Guess what, it was open sesame! Mary said she had a toothache, and opened her mouth for me to examine. I saw a canker sore on her gums that must have been very painful. She had been in pain for two days, and would have probably gone on yelling in pain if no one had stopped to question her. The nurse in charge then addressed her pain. The signs are clear; if someone with Alzheimer's dementia is yelling, there is a reason for it. Please ask questions and investigate further to help them.

Patricia: Paying for a service is part of life. To be able to purchase products or services, and to be able to pay the costs associated with many activities, you need to have the money to pay. Yet, what if your financial circumstances had led you to conserve your income all your life, to stretch every penny? What if money has always been tight, and you have not been able to afford many of life's necessary comforts? This story about Patricia highlights what may occur when a person from a lower income lifestyle develops ADRD.

Each time the hairdresser arrived to bring Patricia to the long-term care home salon, her answer was, "No, I don't want to." It became frustrating for the staff and hairdresser each time she refused. Interestingly, we knew from speaking with her family that she always loved having her hair done at the salon.

Suffering from the later stages of Alzheimer's disease, I knew there was something more to Patricia's choice. I put on my detective hat, and sat down beside her one day and had a little visit. During this visit we reminisced about what it was like going to a hair salon, especially to have our hair done for a special occasion. **(Reminiscing Therapy)** She raved about how much she liked getting her hair done at the salon and told me how she likes having her hair curled. I then asked, "How about we go and get our hair curled at the salon today?"

Surprisingly her answer to this was, "I would like that, but I don't have my purse with me." This comment led me to believe that she had been under the impression that she had to pay for the service. **(Cognitive Concern)** It made sense to me now; all her life she had to pay for things, so she thought she must pay in the long-term care home as well. Instead of informing people she had no money, she just said, "No". Since it was her reality, thinking she needed cash to pay for hair salon services, I knew I could not change her point of view. I had to come into her reality and play along. **(Therapeutic Reasoning™)**

I decided to try something creative. We gave Patricia a hair styling 'coupon' that said, "One free haircut for today only for Patricia." It worked like a charm! With all the "lucky you" statements that followed from the staff, Patricia appeared truly excited to have received this deal! She proudly presented the coupon to the hairdresser and received the services. She understood the meaning of a coupon, as she had used coupons for many years. The value of a coupon was a concept that matched her understanding of the word today. This coupon is now laminated. Prior to each appointment, the hairdresser continues to present Patricia with the laminated coupon. She always smiles in delight when she receives it! We no longer need to work hard at convincing her to get her hair cut.

Chapter Eleven

It may be difficult for those with ADRD to understand why they can no longer live independently, but it's important to keep their point of view intact. Those with dementia need to feel that their reality is still valid or else they may become confused. In some cases confusion can lead to being upset, fear, insecurity, and misunderstanding. Be careful when you're dealing with a person with dementia who can't understand our reality anymore—try to figure out their point of view. Play along; be creative. You will achieve better results and the person you are caring for will be a happier person.

Allie: We all want to feel respected, included, and in charge. These feelings occur when we are asked about our wants, needs, and feelings. It is important to all people that our decisions matter and are taken into account. It is no different for someone with ADRD.

Sitting in the dining room at a long-term care home were two ladies with Alzheimer's disease, Allie and Patty. I knew they would be interested in joining the afternoon Christmas entertainment, so I asked them if they'd like to come and partake. They both agreed excitedly. As we were leaving the dining room, I suddenly heard Allie behind me screaming angrily at one of the care staff.

I turned and quickly accessed the situation. A staff member had taken off Allie's clothing protector bib and put it in the laundry pile **(Trigger)**. As Allie screamed and yelled angrily, "Give it back to me!" the staff member was explaining to Allie, "But you don't need it for the party," and "It's only used for lunchtime."

I understood the staff caregiver's position; she was justified in trying to put the clothing protector in the laundry pile. It was important to her dignity that Allie looked presentable for the party. I also knew that the staff member had approached the situation incorrectly. There was no gentle 'ask' if she could take the clothing protector. She had not given Allie the right to feel she had a choice in the matter. At the moment when Allie's property was removed without explanation or permission, Allie must have felt violated along with many other emotions.

I knew that I had to change the situation immediately, before it got out of hand **(Peacekeeper)**. I said to Allie, "If you would like, I can give you another one that will be much better." **(Therapeutic Reasoning™)** Allie appeared to like what I said, and seemed to respond well to the fact that she had a choice in getting another clothing protector. It did not matter to Allie that she didn't understand the function of the clothing protector. All she understood was she was asked and offered a choice, and her input counted. She agreed with a smile. **(Validation)**

As we started walking out of the dining room again, I decided to start singing Christmas carols to change the mood. **(Activity Therapy/Distraction)** Interestingly, as we walked into the entertainment room, Allie had forgotten all about her anger over the clothing protector incident. The singing distraction and her short-term memory made her forget all about the upsetting situation.

A person with ADRD should be consulted, at least partly in decision-making, to reassure them that their thoughts and feelings count. Caregiving staff and family members should never forget this no matter what stage the person may be in with their condition. If they are treated with dignity, respect, and made to feel that their needs are validated and their decision-making counts even in a small way, this can save everyone involved much aggravation.

Mrs. Kappa: Mrs. Kappa was sitting in a chair outside the long-term care home dining room, with a lap-table securing her down, having her meal apart from the others. She looked extremely preoccupied and sad while mumbling in another language to herself. Her face was creased in an expression of sadness. **(Consider Cognitive Concerns)**

I wondered if Mrs. Kappa had been taken out of the dining room because she had been very disruptive and was causing upset to others. Whatever the case, it was sad to see her there alone. I didn't like seeing her face show misery, so I had to investigate.

Chapter Eleven

Since I did not know Mrs. Kappa, I found out some information from some of the caregivers. I was told that she had been upset and was talking about her children earlier that day. I do know that a person in mid-later stages of dementia, who has grown children, may firmly believe that their children are young and in need of their parent.

Later that day I saw her walking the halls, still looking worried. I had to try something. I went up to her and said in English with conviction and a smile, "Your children are fine." I was holding my breath, but to my happy surprise she looked at me with a worried but slightly relieved face and responded with, "Are you sure?" It surprised me to hear her speak English, but it was wonderful to feel that she seemed to be reassured by my sentence. Once again with a convincing voice and a soft reassuring smile I said, "Yes, I'm sure." **(Therapeutic Reasoning™)** She looked so pleased and thanked me.

Seeing that I had made a small breakthrough, I asked Mrs. Kappa if she was thirsty, and she said yes. I brought her juice, which she drank in seconds. **(Physical)** As I went and filled her glass again, I thought about the symptoms of dehydration, one being a possible headache. Out of curiosity I asked if she had a headache and she touched her temples and said, "Oh yes".

I noticed that Mrs. Kappa was curious about me, a person who seemed to care enough to talk to her and to reassure her. She did the sweetest thing then and there, which still brings tears to my eyes. She reached for my hand, kissed it, and gently said, "Thank you." It's a wonderful thing to love and be loved by people, even if only for a moment. **(Validation)** When you are dealing with individuals with ADRD especially in later stages, take the lead and start searching for the clues to why a person might be acting a certain way. That's when true miracles happen, and that could be how the person with dementia sees it too.

Candice: How would you like it if someone forcibly tried to take you somewhere and you didn't know where you were being taken? I'll bet you wouldn't respond well to that type of treatment, and neither did Candice—she screamed and became agitated when she was being taken without her permission and knowledge. **(Physical, Consider Cognitive Concerns, Triggers)**

A sweet lady with vascular dementia, Candice depended on her long-term care home caregivers to carry out her daily routine. One evening, the staff member in charge started pushing her wheel chair to the washroom, as it was her turn to go. This happened suddenly and without warning, and without a word to Candice about where he was taking her. He simply grabbed her wheelchair from the side and began to push her down the hall. **(Trigger)** Her reaction, as she had no idea where he was taking her, was to put her feet down on the floor to stop him from pushing her.

I could see the confusion on Candice's face, but the caregiver took no notice of it. Because she was resisting, he turned her wheelchair around and started to pull her backwards toward the washroom. This move made Candice feel even more uncomfortable; she started yelling, "I want to be by the window," and became agitated. I could tell she had no idea where she was being taken—a scary feeling for anyone who doesn't understand a situation logically or clearly. **(Cognitive Concern)**

The staff caregiver then tried to explain that he was taking her to the washroom; however, it was to no avail because he was speaking from behind her, not in front of her (which is recommended), and she was unable to see or hear him. Because of the uncertain direction of the caregiver's voice, coming from behind her, Candice could not hear anything but mumbled tones coming from behind her head.

Understandably, Candice became quite upset and started to reach her arms out to grab on to anything, which caused the caregiver to become frustrated so he stopped pulling her and left her in the middle of the hallway. It was a sad sight to see. There she was sitting in her wheelchair in the middle of the hall without

Chapter Eleven

anyone offering help or an explanation. I went over to calm her right away. **(Validation and Interpersonal Therapy)**

As I crouched down in front of Candice trying to console her, she happened to spot the caregiver going by, her face suddenly brightened and she said, "Oh, I know him." I realized and formed a belief that Candice would have had no problem complying with the actions of this caregiver. She knew him; she simply needed to be approached from the front, receive eye contact and have it explained to her that he was going to wheel her to the washroom. She simply needed to know what was going on, as all people do.

As professional caregivers, we are there to care for many people with ADRD. We're there to help make things easier, safer, and more comfortable for them. We're not there to take away their right to make decisions, or to treat them like robots or as tasks. They are human, and should be respected, communicated with, and given choices, like any other person. It sometimes can be easy for busy caregivers to forget to use good care practices. Sometimes, attending a professional development workshop as a refresher, or reading real case study examples (such as this one) can provide us all with important reminders.

Sophia: A mother's love is strong and precious. Mothers provide for their children; whether it is food, shelter, warmth, and guidance, they will make every sacrifice to make sure their kids are healthy and happy. This is where our story starts, with a mother who felt she had to sacrifice herself to feed her child.

Sophia was a sweet woman with mid-stage Alzheimer's disease, living in a long-term care home. Her routine was to come down to social dinners at the home, but she would eat very little. Noticing she was not eating much, the recreation staff tried to determine the cause, and would ask her, "Would you prefer to eat something else?" It was to no avail; with a sweet smile she would always wave her hand to indicate 'no,' and make a facial gesture that indicated she wasn't hungry.

Sophia didn't speak much English so communication was

difficult. Her gestures were clear though; she would sit and stare at her food and her surroundings. Closer to the end of mealtime, she would pack her food to take it home with her. The recreation staff were concerned and wondered if she was getting proper nutrition. Perhaps she was eating her packed up food in her room, at times other than mealtimes. It was not clear what was going on.

I knew we had to do something to understand her and meet her needs. I tried communicating with her using gestures, but in Sophia's case, her English skills were not sufficient for mutual understanding. What to do? Well, we sought and found a volunteer that spoke Sophia's language. Things became very clear once there was translation—we asked her if she was hungry and Sophia said that she was hungry, but she knew that her son who was going to university needed the food more than her. **(Consider Cognitive Concern)** She was saving the food to give to her son who, she thought, was not getting enough to eat while working so hard to become successful. As she answered, it was obvious she was bursting with motherly pride and loving sacrifice.

Unfortunately, most days, Sophia didn't understand that all her children were grown up; they had careers, their own lives, and families. Her son didn't even live in the same city as her. In her "Memory Onion," she thought that she was going "home" to where she had lived for many years, feeding and raising her children. The first approach was attempted by a volunteer, who tried to explain to Sophia that her son no longer went to university, and that he lived in a different city than she did. In addition, the volunteer tried to communicate to Sophia that she did not need to save her food for her son. These explanations were obviously true, but only for those caring for her and our understanding of her reality. Immediately, we began to recognize extreme upset and confusion on her face. Sophia's reality was different—she knew that her son was still in school, and she was still caring for him as a mother to a child. She would not listen or believe the reality the volunteer was attempting to have her enter because of her "Memory Onion." So, all caregivers involved in this situation with Sophia had to change tactics right away.

What Sophia knew all her life, was being a mother, protecting, feeding, and loving her children. We needed to satisfy her reality. **(Therapeutic Reasoning™)** The next time she came down to a social dinner, we explained that we had already boxed up a meal for her son; it was ready for her to take home after dinner, and she need not worry about saving food, because her son's meal was already packed up. We reiterated to Sophia that she could give the food to her son, after dinner. She seemed satisfied with this explanation! The interesting thing was she often forgot about the box dinner for her son when it was time to leave.

> **Helpful Hint:** Reading the stories of individuals with ADRD allows us to better understand and learn how to make their situation better.

In order to provide readers with a viewpoint from a Certified Care Aid in British Columbia currently working in the field, I would like to share some stories that were provided from Erica. Erica has been caring for seniors for 22 years. She has spent ten years exclusively in a dementia care unit and has many stories to share. Here are only a few:

Joe: Joe had been living in long-term care home for about seven years. As he become more and more confused, he would ask the staff every day, "How long have I been here?" **(Cognitive Concerns)** Erica noticed that when staff would say, "Joe you have been here for seven years," he appeared upset. Erica decided she would avoid answering him with the correct number of years he had been living there. Instead she started telling him, "Why don't you stay for one more day? We like having you around." **(Therapeutic Reasoning™)** Then when he agreed while observing her calm smile, she would gently escort him back to his room where he found comfort with familiar things. **(Distraction)**
Sarah: Bathing is a common challenge for many caregivers of

individuals with ADRD. There are several different reasons why a person may refuse to take a bath. Finding out "why" may help you make a choice on the most suitable creative solution. Sarah would refuse to take a bath on the day that she was scheduled. This was mainly because she no longer understood the meaning or reason for taking a bath. In addition, she could not remember how to perform the tasks required in taking a bath. **(Cognitive Concern)** Erica decided to approach her using **Therapeutic Reasoning™** because she knew she enjoyed having her son visit. Erica said, "Sarah, I hear your son might come for a visit today, I'm not sure, but if this is so, it may be a good idea to be ready and all cleaned up before he comes. Let me help you." Sarah reacted with uncertainty and was not entirely convinced. So, Erica added gently, "You see Sarah, I am only able to assist one person for a bath each day and because I know you like to be ready for your visit with your son, I have chosen you today!" Sarah seemed honoured. Erica continued, "The only problem is you can't tell anyone else as they will get jealous." **(Therapeutic Reasoning™)** Consequently, as they were walking down the hall, towards the bathing area, Sarah had a furtive look on her face as she walked past the other residents, confirming to Erica that Sarah did not want others to know the secret. This creative solution worked like a charm on Sarah because she was happy to follow Erica's logic as it allowed her to feel superior, therefore valued and important.

John: Erica noticed that staff members were starting to fear working with John because of his angry ways when they gave him a bath. **(Physical)** At times, there had to be two staff members holding him down and this solution would only make him angrier. **(Cognitive Concerns)** John would begin to use swear language and yell, "stop" at everyone trying to help with his bath. Erica witnessed staff yelling back at him to "stop resisting." They would say, "We have to give you a bath! Stop yelling at us!" Erica stated in our interview, "You might be able to accomplish the work by doing the task this way, but this will certainly leave the

Chapter Eleven

resident feeling very upset during and after the bath and maybe injure him." This bath routine always began with staff approaching him in his room early in the morning saying, "Johnny, it's your bath day!"

Erica wondered if there was a better way to negotiate with John on days he was scheduled for a bath. She decided one day to approach him a little differently. Erica said, "Good Morning John! What a beautiful day! Did you say you were from Sweden? Did they have spas in Sweden where women and men could go to get pampered? What was the name of the spa in your city?" Erica would talk with John first to gain his trust. **(Reminiscing)** They would continue talking while she gently pushed his wheel chair to the tub room. On the way, they sang songs he recognized. When they got to the tub room, Erica recalls John saying, "No, I am not taking a bath!" Erica told me that she felt it was best to treat him "like he was a king" and to make him feel you don't want to hurt him. Erica said, "John, I understand you want to be clean for breakfast. I also know that you hate this machine that puts you in the tub. How about this, I will promise to be as gentle as I can to help you get cleaned up, but I will need your help. Let's do it together. I will go as slowly as I can and if you feel it is too much for you, tell me and I will stop." John agreed. As he was being lifted into the tub, he began to show signs of discomfort. She said to him, "It looks like this is uncomfortable for you? We only have a few more inches to go. Can I continue if I go slower?" Once again he agreed with no swear words. Erica recalled that it appeared as though John enjoyed being treated like he was in control and that he believed that she was going to be gentle. There was no swearing during their visits. Erica uses the term "visit" each time she is required to do a care task with her residents as this has helped her to view the situation differently. She feels that when other care aids look at their tasks as a burden, it does not help matters.

Thanks for sharing your stories, Erica. I wish you much success as you continue on your caregiving journey.

Chapter 12

Being Proactive

"Doing the best at this moment puts you in the best place for the next moment."
Oprah Winfrey

As you become more familiar with the person you are caring for, you will be better able to understand them and avoid situations getting out of control. You will also be able to better determine if a medical issue requires professional medical attention, such as a delirium. Make a doctor's appointment as soon as possible to avoid delaying treatment, or bring the person you are caring for to a walk-in clinic, or emergency department if the walk-in clinics are closed. The longer you wait the more serious the situation may become.

When Is It Time For Professional Support?

If you are suddenly feeling unsafe with the individual you are caring for, due to a violent episode it is best to stay out of reach and do what you can to calm them down. This may include saying nothing and/or leaving the room. For example, if your wife is holding an object that could cause you harm and she is yelling at you to get out of the house because she does not recognize you as her husband, you may want to say to her, "Okay I will leave. I am sorry to upset you." If you try to convince her you are her husband and will not be leaving, this could cause more troubles. In situations like this, if it is safe to leave her alone, it may be best to allow her to have some control. Let her see you take your coat and leave the house. Be sure to take your car, home key, and wallet first. Leaving will allow her the opportunity to calm down. After a little while, come back or try calling her on the phone to ask how she is doing. Her mood will likely become calm in a few hours, or perhaps by the next morning. If this problem becomes a recurring theme at night, here are some possible suggestions. You may consider sleeping in another room, or asking someone else that you both trust stay the nights with you both.

> **Helpful Hint:** Safety comes first!

If you are not sure what to do or say in a particular situation, you many need to try using some of the other coping strategies mentioned in chapter four, such as seeking support from others. However, if you are in a situation where you have tried some creative techniques but are not feeling safe and fear immediate harm to both of you, and nothing you say or do is helping, you may need to call for emergency support such as telephoning a crisis line, the police or even an emergency line like 911.

As mentioned several times already, your safety comes first. Your loved one or client may need assistance such as alterations made with medications that only a medical professional can assist you with. Again, seeking this type of support is not a sign of failure, but rather stepping aside to let those who can make a difference do their part. You did the best up until that point and deserve full appreciation for all your efforts.

I wish I could be there with caregivers in the moment to help with creative coping possibilities in times of distress. Realistically, this is not possible. As an alternative, this book seeks to prepare caregivers as much as possible by offering new insights on how to cope and manage difficult behaviours to the best of their abilities.

When a Caregiver Can No Longer Manage the Care

The ideas and strategies presented in this book may be used as a resource for any caregiver. Opening your mind to the possibility of thinking in a new way and to appreciate that a new paradigm is now in progress surrounding dementia related care practices. By making your best attempts to incorporate some of the behaviour management strategies discussed in this book, you may potentially be saved from experiencing caregiver burnout.

As discussed previously, a caregiver needs to be able to recognize when to ask for and openly accept help. Unfortunately, I have witnessed caregivers who did not accept help when they should have, and instead they asked for support when it was too late to save them from the stress that causes major health problems.

I would like you to take a moment, especially if you are a family caregiver, to think about who might look after your loved one if you become sick? Your family? A hospital? Your government?

As you are no doubt aware, there is a shortage of hospital beds. This is because hospitals are pressed to move people along who no longer need acute (short-term) care. Needing the beds, hospitals are required to move persons with ADRD into more suitable living environments such as back to their home in the community or into a long-term care home. We also know there is a shortage of beds in long-term care homes, particularly in Canada. In many of the communities in Canada, there is a waitlist to move into a government subsidized long-term care bed. These bed shortages need to be considered when you, as a family or paid caregiver, decide it is time to declare that the caregiving role has become too much for you.

> **Helpful Hint:** Consider who will take care of you, if the caregiving role burns you out? It is best to know your options in advance.

In other words, there will be a waiting period that transpires between when you, as a caregiver, decides your task is no longer possible and the actual placing of your client, or loved one, in a setting where more support will be available. Thus, it may be helpful to consider the following series of steps that are involved when placing a person with ADRD in a public or private long-term care home.

The first step is to discuss your concerns with family members and/or a government health authority. The government will more than likely appoint a Case Manager. This Case Manager will assess the needs of the individual, within the mandate of the government health authority and set up a schedule of services to best match the needs of the person with ADRD.

As a family member, making the decision to move your loved one into a long-term care home can be difficult and overwhelming. In Canada, a Case Manager will need to place your loved one's name on the government's subsidized long-term care bed wait list. As detailed above, this move will not happen overnight. You or someone else will need to continue the caregiving role in the home until a bed becomes available somewhere.

According to a report by Ombudsperson Kim Carter released in February 2012 on "The Best of Care: Getting it Right for Seniors in British Columbia (Part 2)," there have been many cases in BC where families have waited between one month up to one and a half years to be offered a bed for their loved one. Sadly, this is a common problem across Canada, not just in BC.

I am sharing this information with you now because often families are not aware of the waiting time that may be involved when a decision has been made to move a loved one diagnosed with ADRD into a long-term care home. To provide an analogy, perhaps you decide to go out for New Year's Eve and plan to call a cab to get home later. If you haven't already experienced waiting for a cab on the busiest night of the year, you will be in for a shock as to how long you will actually have to wait to get home!

It will be unfortunate if you find yourself going through a similar shock regarding finding a long-term care placement for your loved one or client. It is important to consult with a Case Manager before you have reached the point where you are desperate for long-term care support. It may be wise to have your loved one or client placed on the waiting list for government services well before you reach the point of deciding you can no

Chapter Twelve

longer care for the person with ADRD in the home setting. In terms of actually being offered a placement after your loved one or client's name reaches the top of the waitlist, it is an unfortunate reality that families in most communities often do not have the choice of long-term care home location when utilizing the public or government system.

If the family is planning and is able to commit financially to pay the private rates for a care home of their choice, it is important to understand that a vacancy will also be required. Therefore, it is important to plan ahead and make arrangements long before the decision is made to move your loved one or client into assisted living or a private care home. I fully understand how this can all be very complicated. Know that the procedures and rules will vary for each province in Canada. It is best to contact your doctor or local government home health office for more information.

Waiting with your loved one for the call for an available bed in a long-term care setting may be a stressful experience. Families may be hard pressed to get through the waiting period. As previously noted, the wait may extend from one month up to one and a half years. If your family is caught in this bind and the finances can be found, please consider playing someone to help out for a couple of months. Families may feel that watching the bottom line (being frugal with money spent on additional help) is more important than reducing their own personal stress levels. However, I want to remind you if you are in this position that you are worthy and important!

To reiterate, please consider help, even if you have to pay a worker to assist you for a few months. There are several home care companies to choose from. Money spent on help may be in the best interests of all involved during the interim and in the long term. Please don't close down your options for the sake of saving a few dollars. The "rainy day" may be now. Speak to a financial planner who will be able to advise you. You can also bring these concerns to your Case Manager.

> **Helpful Hint:** You are worthy, important, and valuable!

Planning Ahead

As mentioned earlier, future legal document planning, in addition to financial planning, may also help to alleviate some of the shock that may occur down the road if the family has not made adequate arrangements. These plans should include having all legal documents such as Power of Attorney, and Representative Agreements (also known as Power of Personal Care in other provinces) prepared while the person with ADRD remains capable. If all the correct paperwork has not been prepared in advance, it may be very costly to have to go through the court system to set things up after the fact.

In terms of being proactive, you may also want to discuss 'end of life' plans with your loved one. Perhaps a 'living will' document may be drawn up or plans for palliative care formalized. Capturing your loved one's wishes while they remain able to express them will better prepare family members to make decisions should the 'end time' arise. Lastly, although never an easy topic, funeral planning will certainly reduce stress on surviving family members when a death does occur. Making all these difficult plans in advance will reduce stress and pain in the future. Putting these arrangements on your to-do list today will only make your life easier tomorrow.

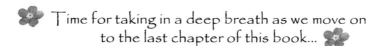

Time for taking in a deep breath as we move on to the last chapter of this book...

Chapter 13

Hopes for the Future

"Hope is definitely not the same thing as optimism. It is not the conviction that something will turn out well, but the certainty that something makes sense, regardless of how it turns out."
Václav Havel

When we are faced with the complications and uncertainty of Alzheimer's disease and other related dementias (ADRD), one reliable common denominator that everyone may count upon is hope. Hope, as Mr. Havel expresses so brilliantly, helps us make sense out of difficult circumstances and find inspiration to search for solutions.

Certainly, there are things we can all do to maintain a healthy brain as mentioned in chapter two; such as eat right, exercise the brain, exercise the body, get plenty of sleep, stay social, and live with minimal stress. But what about those who have already been diagnosed with ADRD? What can caregivers do, right now, to offer daily support? This book was written to provide suggestions for addressing common daily behaviours. Utilizing applicable daily care supports will go a long way to help people who are currently diagnosed with ADRD.

In addition to providing excellent daily supports for persons with ADRD, and as discussed in the Author Prologue at the beginning of this book, a new paradigm is emerging in dementia related care. Using creative non-pharmacological interventions as a first defence to manage behaviours of someone with later stages of ADRD is the foundation of this new paradigm.

John Zeisel, Ph.D., President, Hearthstone Alzheimer Care, Lexington, MA and Paul Raia, Ph.D., Director, Family Support & Patient Care, Alzheimer's Association of Eastern Massachusetts, Cambridge, MA1, together published a study in 1999 called

"Non-pharmacological Treatment for Alzheimer's Disease: A mind-brain approach." In this report the author writes the following:

> *"Emphasizing non-pharmacological treatments linked to our growing understanding of neuroscience, this new vision appears to be sparking the imagination of caregivers, clinicians, designers and others concerned with people living with dementia."*

Yes, I would agree; non-pharmacological treatments have certainly sparked my interest. One of my biggest beliefs is that these new "paradigm" ideas in dementia care will normalize in the imaginations and daily practices of others across the world.

The Future of Dementia Related Care in Canada

In 2012 the World Health Organization (WHO) revealed that Canada is one the countries that does not have a National Strategy for dementia related care. Readers may take a look at The Alzheimer Society of Canada's Dementia Crisis website, a website that asks Canadians to be part of the country's awakening to this disease being a crisis and our need for a plan: www.canadadementiacrisis.ca. Further, for an opportunity to encourage your local member of parliament to push for a National Strategy or plan you can find more information about this on the Alzheimer Society of Canada's website at www.Alzheimer.ca.

In terms of quality care for persons with ADRD in long-term care homes across Canada, the most important contributing factor is adequate staffing levels. Staffing shortages lead to a lack of time available to ensure that resident needs are understood and met. When staff are hurried and unable to take time to provide for the emotional and physical needs of a resident, the quality of care declines, behaviours could arise and the overall health of the residents suffers.

Chapter Thirteen

In addition, the staff members need to be appropriately trained and educated. More opportunities for dementia training needs to be available and offered throughout Canada to ensure all health care professionals across the continuum of care are well-trained in understanding ADRD and to understand a wide range of strategies to manage the resulting behaviours.

From a provincial standpoint pertaining to the province where I currently reside, the February 2012 report, prepared by BC Ombudsperson Kim Carter, is a valuable resource that provides rationale for improvement in overall staffing levels throughout the continuum of dementia related services. The report called "The Best of Care: Getting it Right for Seniors in British Columbia (Part 2)" contains a comprehensive and in depth investigation with 143 findings and 176 recommendations designed to improve home and community care, home support, assisted living and residential care services for seniors.

Further, it was reported that the BC Ministry of Health has yet to develop a planned approach to the delivery of care and services to seniors in residential care who are affected by ADRD. Many recommendations were presented in the Kim Carter report including enhancing dementia and end-of-life care services in residential care. Recommendation number 145 states:

"The Ministry of Health build upon its own BC Dementia Service Framework and work with the health authorities to:
- Develop a provincial policy to guide the delivery of dementia care in residential care facilities
- Ensure that all residential care staff receive ongoing training in caring for people with dementia."

On a positive note, the health authorities in BC have responded to some of the recommendations in the Kim Carter report and the Ministry of Health is currently considering the majority of the Ombudsperson's recommendations. Although it has been and will be a very slow process to see these changes, I remain hopeful. The Ombudsperson will monitor progress that is made on the recommendations and report the results through the office's website at www.bcombudsperson.ca.

A recent positive news story made headlines on June 11th 2013. Janet Brown from CKNW news talk (AM980) published an article called "A different way to treat dementia." It was very exciting to read that the British Columbia Care Providers Association has come up with a new guide that it says will reduce the need for anti-psychotic medications in long-term care facilities. The article states, "The new guide advocates for non-pharmaceutical options such as music and aroma therapies to treat people with dementia." It goes on to say that these methods have been tried in various care homes around the province and one of the facilities had a 25 percent reduction in the use of anti-psychotic drugs.

It has been evident to me that progress has been occurring over the years across Canada in improving dementia care standards. This is certainly positive. However, change does take time. Let's continue to remain hopeful.

Future of Dementia Related Care around the World

In 2011, the World Health Organization released a report titled "Dementia a Public Health Priority." This report addresses the high global prevalence and economic impact of dementia on families, caregivers and communities. The preface of this report indicates:

> *"The report is expected to be a resource that will facilitate governments, policy-makers, and other stakeholders to address the impact of dementia as an increasing threat to global health. It is hoped that the key messages in the report will promote dementia as a public health and social care priority worldwide."*

Chapter Thirteen

Ultimately, my hope for the world is that the devastating effects of ADRD for both the caregivers and those diagnosed will be vanished! In the meantime, since Alzheimer's disease and other related dementias are a worldwide problem, let's hope all countries make a commitment to creating a national strategy that includes better support for family caregivers, better education for paid professionals, a continuum of services to support all stages of ADRD, better public awareness, and funds allocated towards research. Would you not agree that our loved ones deserve it?

Conclusion

I never said it would be easy, I only said it would be worth it."
Mae West

One Last Review

Most days, I need to hear or see things several times before I am able to retain it. If you are anything like me, here is a quick review of fundamentals of this book to assist you in retaining these helpful ideas:

To Crack the Dementia Code…

We first need to realize and accept there is a **Reason for the Behaviour.**

Then put your **Detective Hat** on to figure out reasons **WHY** the behaviour is happening.

To figure out **WHY** you than want to gather the
Ph.A.C.T.S.™:

Ph - Physical?
A - Ask Them!
C - Consider Cognitive Concerns
T - Triggers?
S - Scan the Environment

Then, once the Ph.A.C.T.S.™ have been determined, take off your detective hat since you won't need it anymore and put on your **Creative Hat** to determine helpful creative solutions.

Here is the list of non-drug therapies that have helped me to manage behaviours over the years:

- Validation
- Interpersonal Therapy
- Therapeutic Reasoning™
- Re-Direction
- Activity Therapy
- Music
- Art
- Reminiscing Therapy
- Address Physical Needs
- Make Environmental Changes

Remember the importance of staying in their reality, so that you can properly personalize solutions to do whatever works to keep the peace and keep them happy and calm.

Other Things to Remember:

- Safety first!
- Not all individuals with dementia should be treated the same way; personalized solutions are needed.
- Try to remain calm: If you do become frustrated or lose your temper, know this is common. Regard these instances as a sign that you need some extra support.
- Don't be afraid to ask for help.
- You can't change someone else; you can only change how you respond to the situation.
- Don't be shy to use Therapeutic Reasoning™ if the individual is not able to come to our reality. You are doing this to help not hurt.
- It's okay for you to take a breather and try again in a few minutes.
- Try to be patient; it is the disease at work.

Conclusion

- Do whatever works!
- Be as creative as you like!
- Trial and error.
- Stay positive.
- Keep learning.
- Don't forget to keep your sense of humour.
- **Be sure to give yourself a big pat on the back for all you are doing!**

Afterword: My Final Message To You

Caring for someone with ADRD may not have been in our plans but it has happened. Now all we can do is make the best of our situation. This includes using the creative non-drug therapies and/or approaches suggested in this book and to never stop learning.

Sure, there will be times we make mistakes in our approaches. Let's try not to be too hard on ourselves when this happens. As long as we are learning from our mistakes, committed to continually improving, and doing our best to care for those with ADRD, we will always be moving in the right direction. As we all know, patience when caring for someone with ADRD in not just a virtue, it is essential.

Scientific discoveries are ongoing and we must never forget that we are all doing our best with what we know today and the circumstances we are currently in. Tomorrow will bring new ideas and new discoveries; expect it and continue to stay hopeful.

I am certain that once this book is published; new findings, suggestions and ideas will pop into my head and I will be wishing I could be sharing them with you. Please feel free to stay connected by visiting our website regularly or by signing up for our e-newsletter. You are welcome to join our on-line community where you may access our collection of resources and share your stories with others. This forum allows us to stay in touch, learn from each other and improve in our roles as caregivers.

Please feel free to contact me at any time, if you would like additional support. I will do what I can to assist you with your questions and/or with some creative ideas to manage behaviours for your circumstance. Receiving advice from a third party may help to shine a light on potential unnoticed solutions for your unique situation.

One last time I invite you to take a deep breath as you begin, or continue, your journey as a caregiver for someone affected by Alzheimer's disease or other related dementias with a new perspective and a willingness to try.

 May you never forget the importance of taking deep breaths. Make this last one a great one!

Warm regards,
Karen :)

Citations

About JDNP
www.neurodegenerationresearch.eu/about/

Advanced Gerontological Education – Retrieved on June 10th, 2013
www.ageinc.ca

AISI (2012) Critical Thinking – Retrieved on Apr 20th, 2013
www.education.alberta.ca/teachers/aisi/themes/critical-thinking.aspx

All, Sherrie, Ph.D. (2013) What is Cognitive Reserve?
www.thecognitivereserve.com/Brain_Health_and_Development_Readings/

Alzheimer's Association (2007) Alzheimer's Disease and Other Dementias
www.alz.org/greaterdallas/documents/alzotherdementias.pdf

Alzheimer's Association (2013) Korsakoff Syndrome
www.alz.org/dementia/wernicke-korsakoff-syndrome-symptoms.asp

Alzheimer's Association (2013) Risk Factors
www.alz.org/alzheimers_disease_causes_risk_factors.asp

Alzheimer's Association (2012) Traumatic Brain Injury
www.alz.org/dementia/downloads/topicsheet_tbi.pdf

Alzheimer's Association (2013) What is Alzheimer's?
www.alz.org/alzheimers_disease_what_is_alzheimers.asp

Alzheimer's Association (2013) What We Know Today about Alzheimer's
www.alz.org/research/science/alzheimers_disease_causes.asp

Alzheimer's AUS (2012) Alzheimer's Disease
www.fightdementia.org.au/understanding-dementia/alzheimers-disease.aspx

Alzheimer's AUS (2012) Early Diagnosis of Dementia
www.fightdementia.org.au/understanding-dementia/early-diagnosis-of-dementia.aspx

Alzheimer's AUS (Mar, 2012) HIV Associated Dementia
www.fightdementia.org.au/understanding-dementia/aids-related-dementia.aspx

Alzheimer's AUS (2005) What is Dementia
www.fightdementia.org.au/what-is-dementia.aspx

Alzheimer's Society CAN (2012) Retrieved on Apr 23rd, 2013
www.canadadementiacrisis.ca

Alzheimer's Society CAN (Oct 16, 2012) 10 Warning Signs
www.alzheimer.ca/en/About-dementia/Alzheimer-s-disease/Warning-signs-and-symptoms/10-warning-signs

Alzheimer's Society CAN (2011) About Dementia
www.alzheimer.ca/en/About-dementia

Alzheimer's Society CAN (Mar 25, 2013) Alzheimer's Disease
www.alzheimer.ca/en/About-dementia/Dementias/Alzheimers-disease

Citations

Alzheimer's Society CAN (Sept 27, 2012) Dementia's rising numbers spell trouble for Canada's health-care system
www.alzheimer.ca/~/media/Files/national/Media-releases/asc_release_09272012_newdatarelease_en.ashx

Alzheimer's Society CAN (Jan, 2011) Guidelines for Care: Person-centred care of people with dementia living in care homes framework – Retrieved on Apr 3rd, 2013
www.alzheimer.ca/en/About-dementia/For-health-care-professionals/~/media/Files/national/Culture-change/culture_change_framework_e.ashx

Alzheimer's Society CAN (2010) Rising Tide: The Impact of Dementia on the Canadian Society
www.alzheimer.ca/~/media/Files/national/Advocacy/ASC_Rising%20Tide_Full%20Report_Eng.ashx

Alzheimer's Society CAN (Nov 22, 2012) Lewy Body Dementia
www.alzheimer.ca/en/About-dementia/Dementias/Lewy-Body-Dementia

Alzheimer's Society CAN (Nov 2, 2012) Risk Factors
www.alzheimer.ca/en/About-dementia/Alzheimer-s-disease/Risk-factors

Alzheimer's Society CAN (Mar 25, 2013) Vascular Dementia
www.alzheimer.ca/en/About-dementia/Dementias/Vascular-Dementia?p=1

Alzheimer's Society CAN (Mar 25, 2013) Wernicke-Korsakoff syndrome
www.alzheimer.ca/en/About-dementia/Dementias/Wernicke-Korsakoff-syndrome

Alzheimer's Society CAN (Mar 1, 2013) What is Alzheimer's Disease?
www.alzheimer.ca/en/About-dementia/Alzheimer-s-disease/
What-is-Alzheimer-s-disease

Alzheimer's Society CAN (Nov 10, 2012) What is sundowning?
www.alzheimer.ca/en/About-dementia/Understanding-
behaviour/Sundowning

Alzheimer's Society UK (2013) Alzheimer's Society
www.alzheimers.org.uk/site/scripts/documents.
php?categoryID=200126

Alzheimer's Association USA (2013) What is Dementia
www.alz.org/what-is-dementia.asp

Angelone, Anne, MS (May 23,2013) The Link Between Gut Bacteria, Depression, Anxiety, and Weight Gain
www.primaldocs.com/opinion/the-link-between-gut-bacteria-depression-anxiety-and-weight-gain/

Anonymous, University of Cambridge (Aug 10, 2012). Delirium Increases the Risk of Developing New Dementia Eight-fold in Older Patients
www.cam.ac.uk/research/news/delirium-increases-the-risk-of-developing-new-dementia-eight-fold-in-older-patients

Arch Neurol. 2011 February; 68(2): 214–220.
doi: 10.1001/archneurol.2010.362 - :
www.ncbi.nlm.nih.gov/pmc/articles/PMC3277836/

Barnes, Irene Iris (2007) Musings from a Dementia Unit: Learning from Elders with Alzheimer's– Retrieved on June 2nd, 2013

Citations

Baycrest (Mar 19, 2012) Mild Cognitive Impairment
www.news.baycrest.org/2012/03/mild-cognitive-impairment.html

Behaviour. (n.d.). Oxford Dictionary.- Retrieved June 12th, 2013 from Oxford Dictionaries website
www.oxforddictionaries.com/definition/english/behaviour?q=behaviour

Bookman, Todd (Feb 4, 2013) The Battle Against 'Chemical Restraints' Inside Nursing Homes – Retrieved on June 1st, 2013 from
www.nhpr.org/post/battle-against-chemical-restraints-inside-nursing-homes

Bowlby Sifton, Carol (Feb, 1997) Emotional awareness and emotional memory
www.caot.ca/default.asp?pageID=3699

Brackey, Jolene (2007) Creating Moments of Joy for the Person with Alzheimer's or Dementia: A Journal for Caregivers
Apr 20th, 2013

Brown, Janet (June 5th, 2013) A Different Way to Treat Dementia – Retrieved on June 11th, 2013
www.cknw.com/news/vancouver/story.aspx?ID=1977785

Burke, Darla (Aug 7, 2012) Metabolic Dementia Health line
www.healthline.com/health/alzheimers-dementia/dementia-due-to-metabolic-causes

Canadian Mental Health Association (CMHA) (October 26, 2012) Take Control of Stress
www.cmha.ca/mental_health/take-control-of-stress/

Canadian Mental Health Association (CMHA) (January 31, 2012) What is Stress?:
www.cmha.ca/mental_health/what-is-stress/

Carlson, Ann – Intellectual Property Lawyer (Personal Communication, Jan 10th, 2013)

Carter, Kim (Feb 2012) The Best of Care: Getting it Right for Seniors in British Columbia (Part 2) – Retrieved on June 1st, 2013
www.bcombudsperson.ca/images/pdf/seniors/Seniors_Report_Volume_2.pdf

Center for Disease Control and Prevention (Nov 15, 2012) About CJD
www.cdc.gov/ncidod/dvrd/cjd/

Chestnov, Dr. Oleg, WHO (Apr 11, 2012) Dementia Cases Set to Triple by 2050 but still Largely Ignored.
www.who.int/mediacentre/news/releases/2012/dementia_20120411/en/

Claris Companion (May 18, 2013)
www.clariscompanion.com

Dana, Dr. Daniel (2006) Managing Difference – Retaliatory Cycle – Retrieved on Apr 20th, 2013

Davis, Charles Patrick, MD, PhD (2013) Parkinson's disease Dementia
www.emedicinehealth.com/parkinson_disease_dementia/article_em.htm

Davis, Dr. Justin (Mar 7, 2013)
www.nognz.com

Citations

Deaux, Tori (Aug 4, 2009) Why You Need a Cognitive Reserve (and how to build one)
www.brainfitnessnow.wordpress.com/2009/08/04/why-you-need-a-cognitive-reserve-and-how-to-build-one/

DeMarco, Bob (May 14, 2011) What's the Difference Between Alzheimer's and Dementia
www.alzheimersreadingroom.com/2010/06/whats-difference-between-alzheimers-and.html

Deo, Brian – Music Therapist (Personal Communication, May 26th, 2013)

Department of Psychiatry, University of California, San Francisco (May, 2012) Midlife vs late-life depressive symptoms and risk of dementia: differential effects for Alzheimer disease and vascular dementia.
www.ncbi.nlm.nih.gov/pubmed/22566581

The Digby Courier Column (June 3rd, 2013) Doing What She Taught Me – Retrieved on June 18th, 2013 from:
www.digbycourier.ca/Opinion/Columnists/2013-06-03/article-3266973/Doing-what-she-taught-me

Division of Geriatric, S. John-Addolorata Hospital, Rome, Italy (July 25, 2013) Is there a relationship between high C-reactive protein (CRP) levels and dementia?
www.ncbi.nlm.nih.gov/pubmed/19836632

Doctoral Programme in Music Therapy, Department of Communication & Psychology , Aalborg University (Apr, 2013) Individual music therapy for agitation in dementia: an exploratory randomized controlled trial
www.ncbi.nlm.nih.gov/pubmed/23621805

Douglas, Simon; James, Ian; Ballard, Clive (2004) Non-pharmacological Interventions in Dementia – Retrieved on Apr 20th, 2013 from www.apt.rcpsych.org/content/10/3/171.full.pdf+html

DSM (2013) Mild Neurocognitive Disorder. www.dsm5.org/Documents/Mild%20Neurocognitive%20Disorder%20Fact%20Sheet.pdf

Genova, Lisa (Jul 13, 2007) Book Still Alice (p. 175)

Graham, Judith (May 1, 2013) Does Depression Contribute to Depression? www.newoldage.blogs.nytimes.com/2013/05/01/does-depression-contribute-to-dementia/

Guide to Brain Health (Mar, 2007) Dementia – The Dana Guide www.dana.org/news/brainhealth/detail.aspx?id=9804

Heerema, Esther, MSW (Feb 25, 2013) 9 Benefits of Consistent Caregivers for People with Dementia – Retrieved on May 5th, 2013 from About.com Guide

Hefti, Franz; Goure, William F.; Jerecic, Jasna; Iverson, Kent S.; Walicke, Patricia A.; Krafft, Grant A. (Apr 10, 2013) The Case for Soluble Aβ Oligomers as a Drug Target in Alzheimer's Disease – Vol. 34, Is. 5 www.cell.com/trends/pharmacological-sciences/abstract/S0165-6147(13)00043-6

Hippius, Hanns, MD (Mar 5, 2003) The Discovery of Alzheimer's disease www.ncbi.nlm.nih.gov/pmc/articles/PMC3181715/

Citations

Hippocrates. (n.d.). BrainyQuote.com. Retrieved June 16th, 2013
www.brainyquote.com/quotes/authors/h/hippocrates.html

Hooper, Brenda (2013) StepByStepMediation.com – Contact Made on: May 28th, 2013

Jasmin, Luc, MD, PhD, VeriMed Healthcare Network, and Zieve, David, MD, MHA (Feb 16, 2012) Dementia Due to Metabolic Causes
www.nlm.nih.gov/medlineplus/ency/article/000683.htm

Jasmin, Luc, MD, PhD, VeriMed Healthcare Network and Zieve, David, MD, MHA (Feb 16, 2013) Pick's Disease
www.nlm.nih.gov/medlineplus/ency/article/000744.htm

Java Music Club – Retrieved on Apr 11th, 2013
www.javamusicclub.com/

Jones, Moyra (2007) Gentle Care™: Revised Second Edition- Retrieved on June 10th, 2013

Kazui H, Mori E, Hashimoto M, Hirono N, Imamura T, Tanimukai S, Hanihara T, Cahill L. (Oct, 2000) Impact of Emotion on Memory - Controlled Study of the Influence of Emotionally Charged Material on Declarative Memory in Alzheimer's Disease
www.ncbi.nlm.nih.gov/pubmed/11116776

LaFee, Scott (Apr 23, 2012) Plaque Deposits Alone Do Not Trigger Clinical Symptoms of Alzheimer's, Researchers Find
www.ucsdnews.ucsd.edu/pressreleases/clinical_decline_in_alzheimers_requires_plaque_and_proteins/

Lang, Amanda (Feb 10, 2012) The Power of Why – Retrieved on Apr 20th, 2013
www.harpercollins.ca/books/Power-Why-Amanda-Lang/

Lewy Body Dementia Association (2012) What is LBD?
www.lbda.org/node/7

Lin FR, Yaffe K, Xia J, et al. Hearing Loss and Cognitive Decline in Older Adults.JAMA Intern Med. 2013;173(4):293-299. doi:10.1001/jamainternmed.2013.1868.
www.archinte.jamanetwork.com/article.aspx?articleid=1558452

Link, Amanda (May 29, 2013) Having a Brain Healthy Lifestyle
www.seniorsguideonline.com/blog/senior-health/having-a-brain-healthy-lifestyle#.Ub1GKmxraP8

Manage. (n.d.). Online Etymology Dictionary. Retrieved on June 12, 2013 from Dictionary.com website
www.dictionary.reference.com/browse/manage

Mayo Clinic Staff (Feb 9, 2013) Alzheimer's Genes: Are You at Risk?
www.mayoclinic.com/health/alzheimers-genes/AZ00047

Mayo Clinic Staff (Jan 4, 2013) Alzheimer's stages: How the disease progresses
www.mayoclinic.com/health/alzheimers-stages/AZ00041

Mayo Clinic Staff (Jan 4, 2013) Alzheimer's stages: How the disease progresses
www.mayoclinic.com/health/alzheimers-stages/AZ00041/NSECTIONGROUP=2

Citations

Mayo Clinic Staff (Apr 16, 2013) Causes Definition
www.mayoclinic.com/health/dementia/DS01131/
DSECTION=causes

Mayo Clinic Staff (Aug 15, 2012) Delirium Definition
www.mayoclinic.com/health/delirium/DS01064

Mayo Clinic Staff (July 3, 2013) Huntingtons Disease Definition
www.mayoclinic.com/health/huntingtons-disease/DS00401

Mayo Clinic Staff (May 11, 2012) Parkinson's Disease Symptoms
www.mayoclinic.com/health/parkinsons-disease/DS00295/
DSECTION=symptoms

McClintock, Norah (2000) Volunteering Numbers - Using the National Survey of Giving, Volunteering and Participating for Volunteer Management
www.imaginecanada.ca/files/www/en/giving/n-vm-ca.pdf

Medicalert Foundation (July 28, 2013) MedicAlert® Alzheimer's Association Safe Return®:
www.medicalert.org/products/everybody/package/medicalert-safe-return

MemoVie Group (Apr 30, 2013) Lifelong Exposure to Multilingualism: New Evidence to Support Cognitive Reserve Hypothesis
www.ncbi.nlm.nih.gov/pmc/articles/PMC3640029/

Mount Sinai (Apr 25, 2013) Scientists at Mount Sinai discover a key mechanism for a common form of Alzheimer's disease
www.eurekalert.org/pub_releases/2013-04/tmsh-sam042213.php
Namenda (2013)
www.namenda.com/

Mozes, Alan (Feb 14, 2011) Study Suggests Hearing Loss and Incident Dementia
www.summitmedicalgroup.com/healthday/article/649896/

Office of Communications and Public Liaisons NINDS (June 6, 2013) Dementia: Hope Through Research
www.ninds.nih.gov/disorders/dementias/detail_dementia.htm

Ombudsperson (Feb, 2012) The Best of Care: Getting it Right for Seniors in British Columbia (Part 2) – Retrieved on Jun 5th, 2013
www.bcombudsperson.ca/images/pdf/seniors/Seniors_Report_Overview.pdf

Ombudsperson (Feb 14, 2012) Improving the Care Of Seniors: Ombudsperson Releases Report With 176 Recommendations –Retrieved on May 18th, 2013
www.bcombudsperson.ca/images/pdf/seniors/Best_of_Care_News_Release_final.pdf

Oxford University Press (2013) Disease Definition
www.oxforddictionaries.com/definition/english/disease

Oxford University Press (2013) Syndrome Definition
www.oxforddictionaries.com/definition/english/syndrome?q=syndrome

Citations

Peckham, Charles W. and Peckham, Arline B. (1982) Activities Keep Me Going – A guidebook for activity personnel who plan, direct, and evaluate activities with older persons Apr 5th, 2013 page 3

Perez, Kristin, OTR/L; Proffitt, Mark A., M.Arch; Calkins, Margaret P., M.Arch., Ph (2001) Creating Successful Dementia Care Settings - Volume Three- Minimizing Disruptive Behaviors – Retrieved on May1 10th, 2013

Reasoning. (n.d.). Online Etymology Dictionary. Retrieved on June 12, 2013 from Dictionary.com website www.dictionary.reference.com/browse/reasoning

Reminisce Magazine (2013) – Retrieved on Apr 20th, 2013 www.reminisce.com/

Samadi, Dr. David B. (Oct 11, 2012) Surprising Ways Stress Affects Your Whole Body:
www.foxnews.com/health/2012/10/11/surprising-ways-stress-affects-your-whole-body/

Sando SB, Melquist S, Cannon A, Hutton M, Sletvold O, Saltvedt I, White LR, Lydersen S, Aasly J. (Nov 23, 2008) Risk-reducing effect of education in Alzheimer's disease
www.ncbi.nlm.nih.gov/pubmed/18484674

Senior Gems – Retrieved on Apr 2nd, 2013
www.seniorhelpers.com/SeniorGems
Dr. Carl Rogers (2011) The British Association for the Person-Centred Approach – Retrieved on May 4th, 2013
www.bapca.org.uk/#page

Siviero C. and Cipriani, G. (Feb 15, 2011) Validation Method: an innovative technique for communication that permits a dignified relationship with aged disoriented people and a significant reduction of behaviour disorders. – Retrieved on Apr 3rd, 2013
www.vfvalidation.org/validation/Modulo_SIPI_Cipriani-Siviero2011_italian_english.pdf

Smith, Melinda, M.A.; Wayne, Melissa, M.A.; Segal, Jeanne, Ph.D. (May 2013) Alzheimer's & Dementia Prevention - How to Reduce Your Risk and Protect Your Brain
www.helpguide.org/elder/alzheimers_prevention_slowing_down_treatment.htm

Snow, Teepa, MS, OTR/L, FAOTA Dementia Care and Training Expert Changing the World of Alzheimer`s – Retrieved on Apr 2nd, 2013
www.teepasnow.com/wp/

Southern, Alice (June 2013) Genetic Testing
www.alzheimers.org.uk/site/scripts/documents_info.php?documentID=434

Steckl, Carrie, Ph.D. and Staats Reiss, Natalie, Ph.D. (2013) Reversible Cognitive Disorder – Pseudo dementia.
www.gulfbend.org/poc/view_doc

Stein, Debra (2006) Credibility, Respect, and Power: Sending the Right Nonverbal Signals – Retrieved on Apr 11th, 2013
www.gcastrategies.com/booksandarticles/62/credibility-respect-and-power-sending-the-right-nonverbal-signals/

Tanz Centre for Research in Neurodegenerative Diseases (2012) Familial Alzheimer's Disease Registry www.tanz.med.utoronto.ca/page/familial-alzheimer%E2%80%99s-disease-registry

Taormina-Weiss, Wendy (June 4, 2012) Urinary Tract Infections and People with Alzheimer's disease or Dementia. Disabled World www.disabled-world.com/health/aging/uti.php

Theurer, K., Wister, A., Sixsmith, A., Chaudhury, H., & Lovegreen, L. (In press). The development and evaluation of mutual support groups in long-term care homes.Journal of Applied Gerontology, 1-29. doi: 10.1177/0733464812446866

Turner, Rick; Zeisel, John; Beinart, Phyllis (Nov 3, 2008) Art Therapy for Alzheimers and Dementia www.everydayhealth.com/alzheimers/webcasts/art-therapy-for-alzheimers-and-dementia.aspx

University of California, San Diego School of Medicine (Apr 23, 2013) Archives of Neurology.

Validation Therapy institute website - Retrieved on May 17th, 2013 www.vfvalidation.org/web.php?request=index

Validation Therapy institute website - Retrieved on May 17th, 2013 www.vfvalidation.org/web.php?request=what_is_validation

We Care Home Health Services Caregiver Guide Series (2012) Alzheimer's Disease and Dementia – Retrieved on June 1st, 2013 www.wecare.ca/flipbooks/Alzheimers/index.html

Weeks, Holly (May 4, 2010) Failure to Communicate: How conversations go wrong and what you can do to right them – Retrieved on Apr 20, 2013

What is CTE?
www.bu.edu/cste/about/what-is-cte/

What is Parkinson's
www.parkinson.ca/site/c.kgLNIWODKpF/b.5184077/k.CDD1/What_is_Parkinsons.htm

WorksafeBC (2010) Dementia: Understanding Risk and Preventing Violence – Jun 11th, 2013
www.worksafebc.com/publications/health_and_safety/by_topic/assets/pdf/bk125.pdf

World Health Organization (2012) Dementia – A Public Health Priority.
www.apps.who.int/iris/bitstream/10665/75263/1/9789241564458_eng.pdf

World Health Organization (Apr 12, 2012) Dementia: A Public Health Priority
www.who.int/workforcealliance/media/news/2012/hrhdementia/en

World Health Organization (WHO) (2011) Dementia a Public Health Priority – Retrieved on May 4th, 2013
www.whqlibdoc.who.int/publications/2012/9789241564458_eng.pdf

Yacboski, Wendy (May 11, 2013)
www.weddingceremonyvancouver.ca

Chapter One

Zeisel, John, Ph.D., President, Hearthstone Alzheimer Care, Lexington, MA and Raia, Paul, Ph.D., Director, Family Support & Patient Care, Alzheimer's Association of Eastern Massachusetts, Cambridge, MA1 (1999) Non-pharmacological Treatment for Alzheimer's Disease: A mind-brain approach – Retrieved on May 8th, 2013

Author Biography

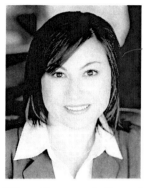

Dementia Consultant and Educator Karen Tyrell, CDP, CPCA is a Certified Dementia Practitioner (CDP) and Certified Professional Consultant on Aging (CPCA). For nine years, she was directly involved with her local Alzheimer Society Chapter in Eastern Canada as a Board member, President for four years and Executive Director for two and a half years. Shortly after moving to the West Coast of Canada in 2009, Tyrell established the Dementia Consulting Company Personalized Dementia Solutions. She passionately supports and educates caregivers through various services and facilitation of workshops such as "Cracking the Dementia Code™" and "How to Maintain a Healthy Brain." Tyrell volunteers in the community supporting charitable and other organizations associated with Alzheimer's and related dementias.

About Personalized Dementia Solutions

Myself and my team of dementia trained coaches work with you to help you understand WHY the behaviours are happening and to come up with creative solutions using a non-pharmaceutical approach. We offer face to face or over the phone/Skype Dementia Consultations. We also offer ongoing Dementia Coaching over the phone to assist you through your day-to-day issues.

Other Services We Offer

Education/Speaking Engagements:

- We provide education for professionals on various topics related to dementia that include a certificate. For example, we provide a two-hour "Cracking the Dementia Code™" workshop. This is available as an in-service or at conferences.
- We offer one-hour workshops for the general public including "How to Maintain a Healthy Brain" or "Cracking the Dementia Code™" for family caregivers.
- Keynote speaking is also available.
- Education may be provided to the entire family in the comfort of their living room or over the phone/Skype, with opportunities to ask questions that are personalized to various situations.

Website:

- Monthly, we produce a helpful News and Knowledge e-newsletter, which includes a section called "Meaning Behind the Behaviours". We provide true stores with examples on how behaviours were managed using creative approaches.

- Helpful information and updates can also be found on our Blog: www.dementiasolutions.ca/blog/
- Learn from others or submit your own question through our Dear Dementia Consultant segment.
- On-line Community Membership is a yearly subscription for both family and paid caregivers which includes receiving discounts on our services and additional information and support.

Dementia Designs™:
We provide recommendations on improving the environment to best support the needs of the individual with dementia. (Includes family residences, retirement residences, hospitals, group homes and long-term care homes.)

Cognitive Massage Therapy™:
We offer the service of creating a personalized schedule with suggestions on activities to keep individuals with ADRD active and stimulated on a daily basis.

Social Media:
Facebook
www.facebook.com/pages/Personalized-Dementia-Solutions/173809079345279 (please like to keep connected)
Pintrest
www.pinterest.com/dementiahelp
Twitter
@Dementia__Help
LinkedIn
www.linkedin.com/pub/karen-tyrell-cdp-cpca/19/b67/b25

To learn more about Personalized Dementia Solutions or to order books, please visit our website at: www.DementiaSolutions.ca

Karen Tyrell, CDP, CPCA
Dementia Consultant & Educator
Personalized Dementia Solutions
www.DementiaSolutions.ca

If you want to get on the path to be a published author by **Influence Publishing** please go to **www.InspireABook.com**

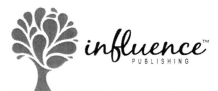

More information on our other titles and how to submit your own proposal can be found at **www.InfluencePublishing.com**

CPSIA information can be obtained at www.ICGtesting.com
Printed in the USA
LVOW06s1728181013

357601LV00032B/2286/P